D0210876

Managing Managed Care II

A Handbook for Mental Health Professionals

Second Edition

Managing Managed Care II

A Handbook for Mental Health Professionals

Second Edition

Michael Goodman, M.D.
Janet A. Brown, R.N., C.P.H.Q.
Pamela M. Deitz, L.C.S.W., M.F.C.C.

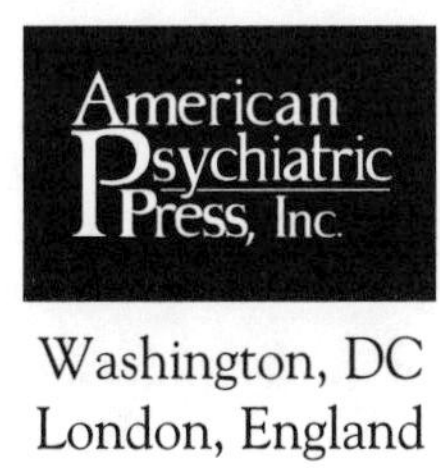

Washington, DC
London, England

Note: The authors have worked to ensure that all information in this book concerning drug dosages, schedules, and routes of administration is accurate as of the time of publication and consistent with standards set by the U.S. Food and Drug Administration and the general medical community. As medical research and practice advance, however, therapeutic standards may change. For this reason and because human and mechanical errors sometimes occur, we recommend that readers follow the advice of a physician who is directly involved in their care or the care of a member of their family.

Manufactured in the United States of America on acid-free paper
99 98 97 96 4 3 2 1

American Psychiatric Press, Inc.
1400 K Street, N.W., Washington, DC 20005

Library of Congress Cataloging-in-Publication Data
Goodman, Michael, 1945–
Managing managed care II : a handbook for mental health professionals / Michael Goodman, Janet Brown, Pamela Deitz. — 2nd ed.
p. cm.
Rev. ed. of: Managing managed care. 1st ed. ©1992.
Includes bibliographical references and index.
ISBN 0-88048-772-0 (alk. paper)
1. Managed mental health care. I. Goodman, Michael, 1945– Managing managed care. II. Brown, Janet, 1945– . III. Deitz, Pamela, 1949– . IV. Title.
[DNLM: 1. Mental Health Services—organization & administration. 2. Managed Care Programs—organization & administration. 3. Disability Evaluation. 4. Documentation—methods. 5. Quality of Health Care. WM 30 G653ma 1996]
RC465.5.G66 1996
362.2′028—dc20
DNLM/DLC
for Library of Congress 96-4743
CIP

British Library Cataloguing in Publication Data
A CIP record is available from the British Library.

Contents

About the Authors

Michael Goodman, M.D., is a clinical psychiatrist in private practice in Beverly Hills and Pasadena, California. He attended Tufts Medical School and completed his psychiatry residency at Northwestern University in Chicago, Illinois. Dr. Goodman has 14 years of experience as a physician advisor with the former California Professional Standards Review Organization and its current successor, California Medical Review, Inc., and is a consultant in managed mental healthcare with treatment programs and practitioner groups participating in newer managed delivery models. Dr. Goodman is an assistant professor at the UCLA School of Medicine, Department of Psychiatry and Neurobehavioral Sciences, Los Angeles, California, and he is also a mental healthcare consultant for the American Medical Association's Doctors Advisory Network, which provides "hands-on" assistance with managed care to members of the American Medical Association.

Janet A. Brown, R.N., C.P.H.Q., is a consultant in quality, utilization, and risk management with psychiatric and medical-surgical, acute and ambulatory, healthcare organizations, all of which are now positioning for managed care. Ms. Brown has 18 years of experience in the evaluation, development, and implementation of effective strategies, systems, and processes to meet federal and state regulations, accreditation standards, and review requirements, as well as managed care and employer/payer information needs. Ms. Brown is the author of *The Quality Management Professional's Study Guide,* now in its 10th edition, and serves as instructor for quality management professionals preparing for the certification exam. She has chaired the national Healthcare Quality Educational Foundation and is the 1995–1996 president of the National Association for Healthcare Quality.

Pamela M. Deitz, L.C.S.W., M.F.C.C., is a psychotherapist in private practice. A graduate of the University of Southern California, Ms. Deitz has continued to work in both agency and hospital settings. Her role as developer and clinical director of an adolescent treatment program heightened her awareness of and interest in the impact of managed care on all clinical disciplines providing mental health services.

Acknowledgments

The revisions and improvements in *Managing Managed Care II* are substantially more than cosmetic. At the same time, this new "handbook" could never have been written without the original "survival guide." Hence, we continue to be indebted to the many individuals who originally encouraged us to forge ahead in what was at one time unfamiliar territory. These pioneers will readily find evidence of their original contributions everywhere. We are also fortunate to have maintained continuity with Editorial Director Claire Reinburg and Editor-in-Chief Carol Nadelson, M.D., at the American Psychiatric Press, Inc. (APPI). Their availability to answer our endless questions personally and their tact and patience when we were teasing our deadline mercilessly are most deeply appreciated. We also thank Ronald McMillen, General Manager at the Press, for deftly guiding us in preparing the sections on software for the automation of impairment-based treatment documentation.

We appreciate the enthusiasm of all those readers of the first edition who "picked up the gauntlet" and began implementing impairment-based documentation in their clinical records. Their experiences using the impairment terminology and documentation method have been invaluable for us. We were also privileged to provide the on-site training for several large mental health provider groups and still have not decided who learned more—them or us. In a hierarchy that is only alphabetical, we thank the many clinicians and administrative staff at Mid Bergen Community Mental Health Center in Paramus, New Jersey, for stimulating our enhancement of the terminology to accommodate longer-term and chronic patients; we are grateful to the Department of Psychiatry, Oregon Health Sciences University, Portland, Oregon, for the opportunity to assess the educational advantages of impairment-based documentation for a multidisciplinary teaching and training center; and we are indebted to the mental health team at St. Joseph's Medical Center in Minot, North Dakota, who had read the "handwriting on the wall" with respect to automated clinical information systems and taught us how we could streamline the teaching process for implementing impairment-based documentation in treatment records.

We are indebted to Joel Yager, M.D., Director of Residency Training at UCLA Department of Psychiatry and Neurobehavioral Sciences, Los Angeles, California, for his relentless enthusiasm and endorsement of our first edition. He also afforded us the opportunity to design a managed care track component in UCLA's psychiatry residency training program. (There is another book waiting to be written on that subject alone.)

We acknowledge the important clinical contributions of David Mee-Lee, M.D., who brought his nationally known reputation and expertise in drug and alcohol treatment to our impairment method. Using his invaluable experience and astute suggestions, we have improved the severity rating qualifiers and patient objectives for the Substance Abuse impairment, and we believe they are now consistent with prevailing drug and alcohol abuse treatment documentation guidelines. We thank Rob Johnson, D.O., Vice President for Medical Affairs at College Health IPA in Costa Mesa, California, who generously gave of his time and demonstrated for us how creative and innovative treatment approaches can spring to life in a delivery model "managed" by the practitioners themselves. We look forward to our continued collaboration with this practitioner group for further outcome studies and treatment research.

We must formally acknowledge our indebtedness to Jeff Bjorck, Ph.D., and his clinical research team. Dr. Bjorck possesses the valuable combination of clinical skill and researcher's logic, and he is giving the impairment terminology the true "stress test." His research notarizes this volume as a true handbook. We also appreciate the dedication of Karen Tanzy, Ph.D., who labored on the tedious task of bringing uniformity to the several hundred individual severity ratings and patient objectives in our database.

There is also a group of talented individuals whose prodigious efforts are only hinted at in this second edition. We are very indebted to the team at Community Sector Systems (CSS) in Seattle, Washington, whose path-cutting work led to the production of a software for automating the impairment-based documentation method. This program module is the first component of a fully integrated mental health information network currently being developed by CSS. We continue to marvel at the perseverance of Dennis Vogt, Executive Vice President of Research and Development at CSS, who delved into the internal workings and deeper layers of our terminology to illuminate the logic embedded therein. He has designed software with data analysis capabilities that are truly astonishing. We must also express our appreciation and gratitude to Gordon Bell, President and CEO of CSS, who has patiently endured detailed debriefings whenever returning from a meeting with one of several dozen managed care organizations or integrated health plans that oversee mental healthcare delivery. This information is very important to us for continuing to meet the documentation needs and expectations of all reviewers and mental healthcare providers.

Preface to the Second Edition

Keeping pace with the evolving and expanding presence of managed care necessitates this extensive revision and enhancement of the previous edition of *Managing Managed Care.* Less than 20% of the original text was carried over to this second version; more than half of the chapters have been retitled, and three of them completely rewritten; two new clinical appendices and a glossary have been added; and all references to pertinent accreditation standards and federal regulations are now current for 1996. The most obvious alteration is the new subtitle, which designates the second edition "A Handbook for Mental Health Professionals" instead of a "survival guide." This "handbook" is intended to be a serviceable reference and a resource for mental health practitioners and for those individuals who will review their treatment services. We hope this edition encourages practitioners to adopt a proactive, informed, and assertive approach to managed care and also to become adept at successfully articulating the clinical rationale for their services. Merely "surviving"—that is, adapting to the recent and unprecedented interposition of managed care between mental health practitioners and their patients—is not enough.

When we wrote the conclusion to the first edition in 1991, we included the following forecast: "A contest over who can deliver the highest quality and most cost-effective care is already under way" (p. 149). We also offered a prediction and affirmed our conviction about the power of the patient impairment profile (PIP) documentation method to give mental health practitioners a winning advantage in the competitive managed care marketplace: "The practitioners 'most fit' to provide convincing evidence for the 'value' of their services will be the ones who survive. The PIP system offers to all mental healthcare professionals the necessary tools for meeting this challenge" (p. 149).

We believe that these predictions have been borne out. Healthcare is now an intensely competitive marketplace industry. Providing value and demonstrating continuous quality improvement are the necessary leverage for winning. Laudatory testimonials from mental health professionals who have manually implemented PIP-based documentation and the enthusiastic response from managed care organizations who have reviewed it were our impetus to produce a more useful handbook for the entire mental healthcare community.

There are four significant modifications that pervade the second edition. First, we no longer use *external* to modify either *review* or *review organizations*. Mental health professionals are now beginning to form their own delivery systems that they promise will also provide quality and cost-effective care. Overseeing or "managing" the care (for quality and value) then becomes an "internal" rather than "external" review function. We now simply use either *managed care review* or *review* throughout the book.

Second, beginning with Chapter 3, we now refer to *impairments* only as a "common-language behavior-based terminology" (instead of the potentially misleading "behavioral language of treatment"), and we specifically define the *patient impairment profile* as a compilation of patient impairments with their severity ratings. The PIP describes "the focus of the treatment."

Third, we have reformulated and further clarified our use of *severity rating, severity level, level of care, intensity of service,* and *treatment setting.* We "unbundled" these terms because their linear "if *x*, then *y*" relationships have turned out to be dubious at best (e.g., the severity of illness/intensity of service utilization criteria notwithstanding). In the rewrite of Chapter 6, we differentiate these terms, define them, and henceforth refer only to *severity rating* instead of *severity level* or *severity level rating.*

Fourth, this edition addresses clinical information needs in mental healthcare beyond those of the individual practitioner. As an inevitable outgrowth of the competitive marketplace phenomenon, professional group practices and provider networks are eclipsing the solo practice model. Managed care organizations, "internal" care managers, practitioner groups, independent practice associations, and health maintenance organizations need an easy-to-use common-language treatment terminology for creating and aggregating meaningful clinical care and outcome data. Managing Managed Care II is written for this wider audience that continues to experiment with these and other managed delivery models—as well as for the individual practitioner who is accountable to them.

The most tangible modification is the addition of the two clinical reference directories (Appendix B [revised] and Appendix C [new]). We have received very favorable progress reports from community agencies and practitioners who are using impairments, severity ratings, and patient objectives to organize their discussions with managed care reviewers. In

Appendix B, we provide qualifiers for each possible severity rating for all critical impairments. As detailed and illustrated in Chapter 6, these severity rating qualifiers prompt the practitioner to supply the most convincing evidence for justifying treatment: patient behavior. These severity rating qualifiers, along with the impairment definitions in Appendix A, give the readers an opportunity to "experiment" with impairments and severities in their very next managed care review. Appendix C is a reference list of patient objectives for the critical impairments. Practitioners can choose to use them "as is" in their treatment documentation or as a model for creating their own. Use of these carefully constructed behavior-focused patient objectives generates very serviceable data for 1) articulating the patient's progress *and* the need for further care, 2) measuring patient outcome, 3) demonstrating the effectiveness of the treatment provided, and 4) documenting the clinical competence of the provider. The format used for these patient objectives is favored by leading nationally based managed care organizations and our clinical outcomes research team.

The extensive changes incorporated into this handbook reflect the integration of many hundreds of comments, questions, suggestions, and observations collected from four distinct professional groups: 1) clinical research psychologists, 2) mental health practitioners and practitioner groups, 3) managed care organizations, and 4) information system and software design and development experts.

Clinical Research

The PIP-based documentation method is being studied by an independent clinical research team, competently headed by Jeffrey Bjorck, Ph.D., of Fuller Seminary's Graduate School of Psychology in Pasadena, California. The first phase of the study consisted of an assessment of the impairment terminology for content validity to ensure its completeness as a set of mental dysfunctions. Four independent groups of expert raters were used, and their recommendations are the basis for the modifications in the impairment terminology outlined below. Two analog studies were then performed in which the raters had access to all 63 impairments and were asked to create the impairment profile for 20 different cases. The true positive hit rate (correctly selecting those and only those impairments for each case) was greater than 90%. These are promising initial results, and replication studies are now under way to validate further the internal consistency and construct-criterion validity of the impairments with DSM-IV (American Psychiatric Association 1994) terminology. The results of these studies to date permit us to endorse the impairment terminology as clinically reliable, comprehensive, mutually exclusive, linguistically concise, and "practitioner-friendly" descriptors for mental health treatment.

Three new "clinical" impairments have been added: Uncontrolled Buying, Uncontrolled Gambling, and Self-Esteem Deficiency. Medical Risk Factor, an important "potential" impairment for concurrent quality and risk management, was added to the impairment lexicon as well. Deficient Frustration Tolerance, Hopelessness, Rage Attacks, Repudiation of Adults as Helpers, and Work Dysphoria were dropped as impairments for two reasons: 1) they more closely resembled explanations for impairments rather than being impairments in their own right, and 2) their behavioral manifestations are taken into account by other impairments.

To ensure mutual exclusivity of the impairments, Paranoia and Delusions were replaced by Delusions (Paranoid) and Delusions (Nonparanoid). Two of the original impairments were a combination of two distinct clinical presentations (impairments), which when combined created a third distinct clinical presentation with its own unique treatment requirements (i.e., Dysphoric Mood With Alexithymia and Marital/Relationship Dysfunction With Physical Abuse). In the service of "cleaner" data elements and research protocol, we separated these "binary" impairments into their true component impairments: Dysphoric Mood, Alexithymia, Marital/Relationship Dysfunction, Physical Abuse Perpetrator, and Physical Abuse Victim. (Any of these may occur in combination with any other.) The original intent of the "with" impairments is still preserved, however, because the treatment plan must take into account not only each individual impairment in a patient's profile but also, where pertinent, the potential ramifications of combinations of certain impairments.

The clinical overlap of the impairments of Hyperactivity and Psychomotor Agitation was resolved by replacing them with Motor Hyperactivity and Anxiety. The "perception" in the impairments of Psychotic Thought and Perception and Psychotic Thought, Perception, and Behavior overlapped with the original impairments of Hallucinations and Delusions. We deleted *perception* from them both and, because psychotic behavior derives from psychotic thought, combined the two to read as one: Psychotic Thought/Behavior. Lastly, the names of several impairments were revised to enhance clarity and be consistent with newer diagnostic terminologies: Inadequate Survival Skills, School Phobia, Paraphilia, and Sexual Dysfunction were renamed Inadequate Self-Maintenance Skills,

School Avoidance, Sexual Object Choice Dysfunction, and Sexual Performance Dysfunction, respectively.

Clinical Practice

We were pleased to have received many valuable and (for us) informative questions, as well as suggestions and endorsements, from mental health professionals who have implemented PIP-based documentation in their treatment records and managed care communications. There is pervasive confusion or, perhaps more accurately, a lack of consensual agreement among mental health practitioners (as well as among and within managed care organizations) regarding commonly used jargon such as *goals and objectives* and *the treatment plan.* We reexamine and reformulate these notions in Chapter 7 and Chapter 8. In the absence of accepted standards that rigorously define the meaning and function of these terms, we propose a "definition standard" for the treatment plan and its essential components. We include the results of our own informal clinical research study on treatment terminology to underscore the extent of the problem and the urgency for remedying it.

Many of the questions raised by clinicians about the PIP documentation method stemmed from this endemic confusion over terminology. Although frequently used in mental health documentation and managed care review, these treatment terms are not rigorously defined (nor do they appear to be systematically taught). We concluded that a glossary was needed for the second edition as part of our commitment to establish a common-language terminology for all clinical documentation, including treatment plans and managed care reports.

We received many questions about patient outcome and outcome studies, particularly in regard to their use for developing clinical standards and practice guidelines for mental healthcare, and those concerns are addressed in the appropriate chapters. Because outcome now encompasses much more than just a change in patient behavior, the term *outcome* in *patient outcome objective* was dropped, and we now refer only to *patient objectives.* Chapter 10 was entirely rewritten to present our informed predictions about "Managing the Future of Managed Care." This title is perhaps a bit misleading because with the phenomenal development of the information superhighway, the "future" is moving ever closer to "now," and outcome management, value management, and information management are "now" the responsibilities that mental health practitioners need to embrace. Finally, the single most frequent inquiry we received was about software to automate the PIP-based documentation method. We are pleased to report that such a software (PsychAccess Clinical Information System) is now available. PsychAccess is introduced conceptually in Chapter 8 and described more fully in Chapter 10.

Managed Care Review

We have reviewed the information requirements of more than a dozen of the largest nationally based managed mental healthcare organizations in the country. We frankly were astonished to learn the number of different ways that (what we believe to be) identical clinical information could be requested from practitioners. The treatment plan model for a definitive mental healthcare treatment plan we propose in Chapter 8 is a synthesis of managed care documentation requirements, accreditation standards, federal guidelines, and what we believe will enable practitioners successfully to compete and "win" in a managed care setting. Needless to say, none of the above-referenced organizations or agencies bear any responsibility for what we have fashioned. In Chapter 10, we also assert our recommendation that a national standard for mental health treatment documentation, including guidelines for "the treatment plan," be adopted by the mental health profession. We hope this second edition will spur movement toward this goal.

We must mention a very intelligent group of fourth-year psychiatry residents who presented us with a concern that clarified the most critical aspect of "the treatment plan problem." We have intuitively known it and understood it but had never formulated it quite so clearly and succinctly as they did. Here is the question the group raised: "Whose treatment plan is it—the patient's or the practitioner's?" The answer to this question embodies the pivotal shift practitioners need to make for successfully and convincingly "talking managed care talk." Managed care has turned its focus of attention away from "How are you managing the patient?" and instead now wants to know "How is the patient managing?"

Information Management Systems

The designers and developers of the architecture and software for automating the PIP documentation method illuminated powerful language links between the impairments, severity ratings, goals and objectives, and (potentially) the practitioner interventions. In Chapter 8, we introduce the concept of *behavior links* between these elements of the PIP method (impairment, severity, goals and objectives, and interventions) for developing a complex relational database for clinical outcomes research. When selecting severity rating qualifiers for an impairment (Appendix B), the practitioner provides patient behaviors to corroborate them. Similarly, patient objectives require the patient to verbalize or demonstrate certain behavior to consider them met or completed. In Chapter 10, we suggest the rich potential of these language links for outcome research and other clinical investigation that can provide answers to some of the most hotly contested issues in mental health treatment.

"Individual Psychotherapy Interventions"—the original Appendix B in the first edition—has not been included in this edition. Although perhaps appearing to be detailed and comprehensive at the time, these interventions were not discretely measurable or sufficiently descriptive of the actions taken by practitioners that we now refer to as "practitioner interventions." For example, "establish a therapeutic alliance" is not a practitioner intervention as we view the term currently (it is actually closer to a patient objective). A positive working relationship between the patient and practitioner in fact is the *result* of particular activities (actions) or techniques that the practitioner believes will facilitate the patient's participation in the therapy process (e.g., validate feelings, clarify the nature of a symptom, mobilize the patient's affect).

An interim "working model" for categories of practitioner interventions is offered in Chapter 8 and will, in fact, be the basis for our next clinical documentation research project. Our task is to describe the interventions as quantifiable practitioner behaviors. We hope to establish meaningful links to the patient objectives (and in turn to the severity ratings) to compare, for example, which interventions are the most effective for a particular impairment or which practitioners who provide the "same" interventions achieve the best result (i.e., the best outcome). We hope to be ready to include a definitive set of practitioner interventions in the third edition.

More than a decade has passed since the ship of private practice mental health began to run out of traditional indemnity insurance fuel. At the time, the entire enterprise appeared to be sinking . . . and those practitioners determined to survive unlashed the lifeboats and set themselves adrift in the unfamiliar and ominous-looking waters of managed care. In Chapter 10, we identify and discuss the converging currents of change that will be carrying the intrepid survivors into the future. We hope this second edition impels mental health practitioners to take charge of their craft and perhaps even take the lead on their way to the as-yet unknown destination of healthcare. One satisfied reader of the original survival guide wrote that "this guide is a lifeboat. . . . it is saving us from drowning in managed care and managed care paperwork." If the analogy holds, and the first edition survival guide was indeed the lifeboat, then we hope that these pages are its sails.

Chapter 1

Introduction

Just being a competent therapist today is not enough to keep one in his or her job. If the title of this book has at all enticed or intrigued you, it is because of your awareness of the increasing demands being made on mental health professionals to convey information about treatment services to reviewers who want to know about them and to future customers who may wish to purchase them. Having to justify one's treatment services to remain in business is one of the most delicate and fiercely debated issues in mental health today. Diametrically opposed professional, political, economic, social, and ethical points of view, coupled with a conspicuous absence of semantic consistency regarding concepts such as "quality care," will no doubt perpetuate this complex controversy into the foreseeable future.

We, the authors, have made a deliberate effort to avoid entering into this heated fray. It is not our intent to take sides in the controversy or assign any blame. What we hope to do in this book is 1) clarify for the reader the issues of practitioner accountability as they relate to both reimbursement decisions and quality monitoring, and 2) introduce an effective proactive response to a current reality that according to all predictions is not going to go away.

The evidence indicates that the American healthcare system is indeed in a crisis. Healthcare in the United States is the most expensive in the world, and yet life expectancy is shorter than in 18 other countries, and infant mortality is worse than in 21 other countries (United Nations 1994). Healthcare expenditures in the United States have surged from $42 billion in 1965 to more than $900 billion in 1994, and it is estimated that in the absence of some radical change in healthcare spending, total healthcare costs will approach $1.7 trillion by the year 2000 (Congressional Budget Office 1995).

The tension in the private sector is particularly acute. Employers are now watching their healthcare spending devour ever larger portions of their profits. In the 1960s, health benefit costs were less than $500 a year per employee. After two decades of cost hikes for health benefits that consistently doubled general inflation, United States employers' overall health benefit costs were an average of $3,741 per employee in 1994 (Foster Higgins 1995).

The increase in costs for mental healthcare services in particular is even more staggering. In 1980, the total cost for mental health and chemical dependency treatment was $35 billion. In 1987, mental health costs comprised about $60 billion, and since then the rate of increase for mental health costs exceeded the rate for healthcare expenditures in general. To illustrate this point, in 1987 the average benefit for mental health and substance abuse coverage cost per employee was about $163. In 1992, it exceeded $400 per employee (Cooper 1994).

A precipitous slashing of coverage for mental healthcare services and, in some cases, the elimination of mental health benefits altogether were unfortunate early responses by a number of employers and insurers to these rapidly escalating costs. But even with such radical measures, the spiral of spending has shown little or no sign of significantly abating. This underscores the urgency with which government and big business are seeking new ways to contain healthcare costs and spend healthcare dollars more effectively.

Managed care is growing by leaps and bounds, not because mental health professionals and patients have fallen in love with it, but because employers, who have become dissatisfied with the skyrocketing costs of fee-for-service care, are hopeful that the promise of predicted savings through management of the care can be achieved. In *The Profit Motive and Patient Care,* Bradford H. Gray (1991) commented that for the time being healthcare professionals will be living through "an unplanned national experiment to see how much medical care can be managed through the use of incentives and review mechanisms" (p. 262). Providing incentives to practitioners to discount their fees and join preferred provider organizations or health maintenance organizations—in return for perquisites such as increased patient referrals and prompt reimbursement—is another form of medical care management that will not be addressed here. How to make one's way through the maze of myriad preferred provider organization networks and health maintenance organizations is the subject of another book that needs to be written. Our book is intended to help mental health professionals keep afloat in the swell of these "managed care" review mechanisms and, at the same time, help independent practitioners and practitioner groups develop their own internal quality management mechanisms.

The term *managed care* has unfortunately been diluted and misused, and there is no longer consensual agreement on the meaning of this term. In its broadest definition, managed care is any patient care that is not determined solely by the provider. *Managed care review* is a general term for any group or organization that examines or scrutinizes healthcare treatment services. Some managed care review organizations, in fact, appear to manage only the immediate expense of care, at times without any consideration of possible long-range costs, quality, or risk. There are other managed care organizations that do undertake the total management of the patient's care, from wellness through chronic illness. Some of these "health maintenance" or "preferred provider" organizations utilize vertically integrated systems of care delivery that allow patients to traverse a variety of levels of care (e.g., hospitalization, residential treatment, day treatment, intensive outpatient therapy, medication management).

Managed care review asks psychiatrists, clinical psychologists, clinical social workers, and marriage, family, and child counselors to justify the necessity for, and demonstrate the effectiveness of, their treatment services. Organizations managing mental healthcare benefits may utilize any of these disciplines to provide the same-coded treatment service. (In this book, we do not "take a stand" on these practices that may or may not affect the quality of care being given.) Nevertheless, all of these professionals are subject to preauthorization and concurrent review for quality. Presently, most clinical training programs for these disciplines do not provide adequate preparation for surviving in this healthcare crisis by meeting these increased accountability requirements. Chinese calligraphy for the word *crisis* is a combination of two Chinese characters: "catastrophe" and "opportunity." In the face of the catastrophe, we saw an opportunity to create a treatment documentation method for not only surviving but, more importantly, for continuously improving quality as well.

In Chapters 2 and 3, we provide an overview of the historical development of managed care and quality review. In the remaining chapters, we take the practitioner step by step through the managed care review process and introduce a method for responding to the various questions posed by reviewers. We also propose a standardized treatment documentation method for all mental health clinical records. This documentation method complies with current requirements for medical recordkeeping and at the same time provides efficacious clinical data for all review functions. Standardized clinical records will yield a rich resource of treatment information (a database) for clinical research and the development of practice guidelines. The standardized documentation method we describe also fulfills the newer requirements now being finalized for the totally automated (computerized) treatment record (Medical Records Institute 1995).

That this current state of affairs may be quite irritating to the busy mental health professional who wishes to devote more time to direct patient care, we do not disagree. At the same time, we have decided to follow the lead of the oyster, which, "when irritated by a grain of sand, makes a pearl." We hope that this book contains some pearls that will help you, the practitioner, manage the review process a bit more comfortably and with slightly less irritation.

Chapter 2

The Public Demand for Practitioner Accountability

"Your services are subject to continued review."

Prior to the first federally mandated professional standards review organization (PSRO) in 1972, the primary responsibilities of healthcare providers were to diagnose, to treat, and, above all, primum non nocere *(to do no harm). In this chapter, we survey the broadening of the healthcare practitioner's duties from private responsibility to public accountability. With the implementation of the PSROs, accountability for utilization of healthcare services became a requirement for reimbursement. The Peer Review Improvement Act of 1982 mandated both utilization and quality review and, for the first time, required Medicare providers to release patient information to a peer review organization (PRO) for* private *review. Private payers could now initiate review prior to payment—hence the feverish proliferation of external review organizations, managed care businesses, and case management companies. These organizations all ask questions now about the medical necessity and quality of healthcare services—questions that most mental health professionals have never been trained to answer.*

The Babylonians were among the first people to develop a systematic practice of healthcare. Their writings as far back as 1600 B.C. include instructions for specific recipes of herbs to treat certain conditions. Occasionally, treatment was overseen or administered by magicians who might also drive out the demons responsible for the afflictions being treated. It was to be another 11 centuries, however, before the quality of healthcare was identified to be the designated responsibility of its practitioners. An oath of physician responsibility attributed to Hippocrates in the 5th century B.C. states:

> I swear by Apollo, the physician, that according to my ability and judgment . . . I will follow that method of treatment which I consider for the benefit of my patients, and abstain from whatever is deleterious and mischievous. Whatever in connection with my professional practice or not in connection with it, I may see or hear in the lives of men, which ought not be spoken abroad, I will not divulge. (Hippocrates as quoted in Goold 1995, p. 299)

For the following 24 centuries, practitioner accountability for the quality of healthcare services was understood and accepted as the practitioner's internal professional sense of moral and ethical responsibility. The established duties of healthcare providers were to diagnose, treat, and, above all, "do no harm" (an axiom attributed to the Hippocratic oath but in fact coming from another Hippocratic work, *Epidemics*).

Within the last 25 years, however, the responsibility for the quality of healthcare services has been significantly redefined for practitioners and, in fact, has been considerably expanded. As a result, today's healthcare practitioners are finding an alarming number of work hours consumed by the demands of utilization and quality review—hours that in the past had been available for direct patient care. How this came to be is a tale of the transformation of medical care and medical information from "private practice" to the public domain.

The first half of the 20th century witnessed initial efforts on the part of healthcare practitioners to monitor the quality of their own peers internally. In 1910, Dr. Abraham Flexner released a study of the quality of medical schools in the United States that stimulated the elimination of "diploma mills." Three years later, the American College of Surgeons was formed as an accrediting body, generating operational standards for medical education and performance. Simultaneously, internal monitoring of healthcare practices was gradually undertaken by state licensing boards and the various city, regional, state, and national medical associations or societies to which healthcare practitioners typically belonged. State licensing boards and medical associations, however, have been characteristically reactive—that is, investigating legal actions taken elsewhere or complaints made by others directly to them concerning a particular practitioner.

In 1952, the Joint Commission on Accreditation of Hospitals—now the Joint Commission on Accreditation of Healthcare Organizations—succeeded the American College of Surgeons as the responsible organization for monitoring compliance with defined operational standards. Since then, the notion that healthcare practitioners are individually and internally responsible and internally accountable for the quality of patient care has been challenged and subsequently redefined. The precedent for institutional liability for the quality of medical care provided by physicians was expanded in the 1965 judicial decision *Darling v. Charleston Community Memorial Hospital.* In this decision, the hospital was held liable for direct duties owed to the patient, for the quality of medical care provided, and for breach of its duty to protect the patient because the hospital knew, had reason to know, or should have known of incompetence by an independent physician.

In 1972, amendments to the Social Security Act mandated the establishment of professional standards review organizations (PSROs), heralding a new level of external professional accountability for the cost, quality, and appropriateness of healthcare services (Social Security Amendments 1972).

In hospital settings, the quality assurance department had originally functioned only peripherally to maintain Joint Commission accreditation. In the 1982 judicial decision *Elam v. College Park Hospital,* the ultimate legal and fiduciary responsibility for the quality of healthcare was placed on the governing body. As a result, *quality improvement*—a term that has replaced *quality assurance* and more clearly communicates the purpose of such activities—moved from the basement into the boardroom. Also in 1982, the Peer Review Improvement Act replaced the PSRO program with the new *utilization and quality control peer review organization* (now shortened to PRO) and for the first time required Medicare providers to release patient information to a PSRO or PRO for private review (Tax Equity and Fiscal Responsibility Act of 1982). This pivotal piece of legislation also opened the door for private payers to initiate review prior to reimbursement. The result was a feverish proliferation of external review organizations, managed care businesses, and case management companies, all of which were asking questions about the medical necessity and quality of healthcare services. Depending on the answers they received, these external reviewers and third-party payers had now been given the legal right to reduce reimbursement significantly or to deny reimbursement totally for those services.

The breadth of practitioner accountability has continued to expand since the implementation of the Medicare Prospective Payment System (PPS) (Title VI of the Social Security Amendments) in 1983. The PPS utilizes the patient classification system of diagnosis-related groups (DRGs) originally devised by John Thompson and Robert Fetter at Yale in 1975 (Fetter et al. 1980). The DRGs classify patients into at least 475 categories based on diagnoses, procedures (e.g., surgery), and comorbid conditions. The PPS replaced the charge-based retrospective payment system for all but a few classes of hospitals. Among those exemptions were psychiatric and alcohol and other drug abuse treatment hospitals and, on application, psychiatric and alcohol abuse units in general hospitals (Federal Register 1983).

At about the same time, and in response to spiraling costs and concerns about the necessity of mental health services, employers reduced their cost of healthcare by restricting patient access to psychiatric and chemical dependency services. This early "managed cost" model has largely been replaced by a "managed benefits" system, which features discounted fee-for-service networks controlled through utilization review. More recently, utilization management has been coupled with continuous assessment of the quality of the provider network. In the near future, managed behavioral care will concentrate on "managed outcomes" (see Chapter 10). As a result of these developments, mental healthcare practitioners have now come to find themselves evermore pressed to respond to questions posed by a medically sophisticated and financially savvy consumer-payer public that wants to know about the quality and cost of healthcare services being purchased.

It is now a prevailing belief that medical knowledge and the activities of its practitioners belong to the community. To this end, a national data bank designed to capture aberrant practices and behaviors of physicians, dentists, and osteopaths was congressionally mandated in 1986 (Healthcare Quality Improvement Act). The Medicare and Medicaid Patient and Program Protection Act of 1987 expanded the reporting requirements to include podiatrists, clinical psychologists, dentists, and essentially any other licensed independent practitioner. The National Practitioner Data Bank is a computerized compilation of disciplinary actions and malpractice payouts against independent practitioners nationwide. Health maintenance organizations (HMOs), group or prepaid medical practices, hospitals, state medical licensing boards, and professional societies that conduct peer reviews to improve quality, as well as liability insurers and individuals and their attorneys, have data bank reporting and querying responsibilities and rights.

Further, the Joint Commission is now actively involved in the development and implementation of its Indicator Measurement System (IMSystem) (Joint Commission on Accreditation of Healthcare Organizations 1995). These clinical performance measures are specialty-specific standards of care with data-driven thresholds of acceptability based on patient outcome. The Joint Commission plans to have on-line access to this set of clinical (as well as other organizational, financial, and administrative) data to facilitate ongoing and concurrent measurement, assessment, and improvement of the quality of healthcare. A 10-year schedule is projected for the medical specialties, and it is to be divided into three phases: 1) obstetrics and anesthesia (Phase 1); 2) cardiovascular, oncology, and acute trauma (Phase 2); and 3) surgery, mental health, and long-term care (Phase 3).

Likewise, the National Committee for Quality Assurance, an HMO accreditation organization, has worked with employers to release the second draft of a set of performance indicators—the Health Plan Employer Data and Information Set (HEDIS 2.0 and 2.5)—which payers can use to compare many different provider organizations (National Committee for Quality Assurance 1993/1995).

Thus, as healthcare and the documentation of healthcare services continue to "go public," so too do the behavior and thought processes of its providers. The once-held belief that "healthcare is healthcare is healthcare" has been dispelled as a "Merlin's myth," challenged by consumers and payers whose faith in the uniform quality of healthcare has been eroding and corroding over time. Unless mental healthcare practitioners can articulate what they are doing for their patients and also convincingly explain why they are doing it, purchasers and providers are going to be increasingly unwilling to pay for their services.

Mental healthcare providers must understand what managed care reviewers need to know, and they must have a means of communicating their response to be reimbursed for their services. The intention of reviewers is not to doubt the clinicians' expertise or their capacity to make good clinical decisions. Reviewers need to know why treatment decisions are made. Practitioners are being asked to articulate their clinical rationale for the recommended treatment, and, for the first time, to provide the supportive, convincing clinical evidence that is the basis for that treatment decision—what is known as "articulating the process of care." Unfortunately, clinicians are not systematically educated about the value of articulating and documenting their own (usually intuitively accurate) thought processes. Instead, they are trained to make the expedient, although tunneled, leap from diagnosis to treatment (as articulated by Hippocrates circa 500 B.C.) with nary a sideways glance at other treatment choices and alternative care options that have become the focus of today's managed care reviewers.

Managed care review at present is often experienced by the clinician as an intrusion—an invasion by an inquisitor reviewer who challenges not only the practitioner's authority but also his or her historical right to operate in private.[1] In fact, managed care review is a request for information to justify what the clinician already knows to be true. It is not necessarily the treatment decision that is being questioned; rather, it is the expert's clinical rationale for that decision that is being examined. Mental health professionals who are trained to ask questions in order to explain the thinking, motives, and behavior of others are now being asked to explain their own thinking and motives in treating their patients.

Managed care review has become an increasingly cumbersome and time-consuming onus on the mental healthcare practitioner. The *impairments* introduced in this book were developed to alleviate this burden. It will be repeated throughout the book that impairments comprise a behavior-based treatment terminology and are not meant to compete or conflict with DSM-IV (American Psychiatric Association 1994) nomenclature. (More will be said about this in Chapter 4.) Dialogue with quality management consultants, third-party payers, and managed care organizations confirms the dire necessity for terse, objective, behavioral de-

---

[1]This conflict is graphically conveyed in the title of an article that appeared in the *American Journal of Psychiatry*: "Psychotherapy Research Evidence and Reimbursement Decisions: Bambi Meets Godzilla" (Parloff 1982).

scriptors of psychiatric patients and the care they receive. Although this insistence on objectification and quantification may offend the sensibilities of those dedicated to the art (and perhaps mystery) of mental healthcare, the posture of the payers appears to be this: if the clinical necessity and outcomes of mental healthcare services are too elusive to measure, then they may well be too elusive to pay for (J. Brown 1995).

Nearly three decades ago, Lawrence Weed (1969) prophesied that "the economic and organizational aspects of medical care, to a far greater degree than students are presently aware, will determine the quality and quantity of care they will be able to deliver" (p. 122). We are now there. The purpose of this book is therefore twofold: 1) to clarify for the mental health professional what reviewers need to know, and 2) to introduce a behavior-based treatment terminology as the basis of a method for effectively and efficiently responding to managed care reviewers and accreditation organizations and to nationwide concerns for quality and value of, and access to, the healthcare product.

Chapter 3

The Need for a Common-Language Treatment Terminology

"Are your services medically necessary?"

There is a diversity of mental healthcare services and an equally diverse, variously trained admixture of managed care reviewers. Current methods of treatment documentation do not effectively communicate the clinical rationale for prescribing particular mental healthcare services. The omnipresent "patient problem list" is inadequate for communicating what reviewers need to know before authorizing reimbursement for services. This situation argues for a common language of readily understood behavior-based patient dysfunctions.

Review of the clinical necessity of mental healthcare services historically began at the hospital level and then only after treatment was well under way or completed. In the mid-1970s, "external review" of patients receiving inpatient psychiatric or chemical dependency services took the form of either "request for additional information" letters to the practitioner or retrospective chart review. In 1988, only five million people with indemnity insurance had their mental healthcare reviewed by case managers. By 1994, the number of insured Americans enrolled in some type of managed behavioral health program had grown to more than 100 million (Oss 1994). Managed care is the delivery system that will also carry Medicaid into the next century. Of the 33.6 million Americans enrolled in Medicaid in 1994, 23% were in managed care programs. This represents a 200% increase since 1985 (Hearn 1994).

In our experience in southern California, more than 80% of private psychiatric inpatients now require certification or authorization for hospital services prior to admission, and their cases are then concurrently reviewed for medical necessity at least weekly. Preauthorization and concurrent review for outpatient mental healthcare services are becoming increasingly common as accountability broadens from inpatient facilities to the practitioners' offices. Quality of care is now being assessed by insurers, employers, managed care organizations, review organizations, accrediting agencies, and, most recently, practitioner groups themselves. The knowledge that this monitoring is occurring and that it is directly linked to reimbursement for treatment services has indeed succeeded in getting the practitioners' attention.

Disturbingly, the individuals and agencies charged with obtaining this information represent multifariously vested and diverse interest groups. Further, the reviewers themselves possess widely varied (and in some cases no) mental health clinical backgrounds. To complicate the problem, third-party payers and managed care organizations approach mental healthcare providers with far from uniform standards for what constitutes quality treatment of mental and substance abuse disorders. At the same time, the responsibility and accountability for the quality of mental healthcare services have been extended and redefined by the Joint Commission on

Accreditation of Healthcare Organizations to include all the disciplines that may treat mental disorders primarily and have an impact on their care secondarily. This, of course, includes any billable or potentially billable mental healthcare service.

The confusion between quality of care, cost of care, standards of care, and justification for care understandably creates a baffling state of affairs for the mental healthcare practitioner—because of the ongoing debate as to just what ultimately constitutes quality mental healthcare. (An answer to this question is offered in Chapter 10.) Traditionally, medical school curricula have placed great emphasis on training physicians to provide "high-quality" care—that is, care that offers available services within accepted standards, utilizing all state-of-the-art technologies and generating clinical data from that care to make further scientific advances in the treatment of disease. Also, high-quality care has been the unquestioned expectation, requirement, and demand of the buyer of healthcare services. As recently as the mid-1970s, quality healthcare was based on two precepts—"doctor knows best" and "spend whatever it takes." However, the cost of such "deluxe care" is now prohibitive. The increasing elderly population, the constant (and increasingly expensive) technological progress, the public demand for quality (and concomitant expensive malpractice settlements), and the fierce competition for the healthcare dollar (advertising) are guaranteed to propel healthcare costs yet higher.

To measure and assess the quality of patient care, one must examine a number of dimensions of the care:

1. Is the care *appropriate* (i.e., clinically necessary) for the condition?
2. Is the provider *competent* to provide that care?
3. Is the care *effective?*
4. Is the care *cost efficient?*
5. Is the care *accessible* and *timely?*
6. Is the care *coordinated over time?*
7. Is the care *safe?*
8. Is the patient *satisfied?*

These are questions that mental healthcare practitioners may have never asked or been asked before.

When faced with a managed care review, the practitioner currently has no idea which of these parameters of quality are being monitored. Even when the practitioner does know the parameter—for example, "Are your services medically necessary?"—the puzzlement continues because most organizations formulate their own idiosyncratic definitions and criteria for these terms. Clear-cut operational definitions are lacking. In the broadest context, clinical care is "appropriate" when the benefits outweigh the risks and are worth the cost; the care may be "medically necessary" if it is required to preserve life or achieve a specified level of function, comfort, or appearance (Eddy 1992). Disagreement arises, however, when deciding to what lengths one goes to try to preserve life and determining what specific level of function, comfort, or appearance one seeks. Interestingly, practitioners and clinical records are not the only data resources being utilized to assess quality of care. A growing number of large employers are asking health insurers and prepaid healthcare plans to ensure the quality of care based on whether the *patients'* expectations of treatment were met (patient satisfaction).

A common language of clinical data elements that is readily understood by all parties concerned is desperately needed. Ideally, this is a terminology that clearly communicates both the reasons for treatment and the thought process (the clinical rationale) concerning the proposed treatment services. This terminology must be easily understood and interpretable both by the professionals with multiple levels of clinical expertise who are documenting the treatment and by the equally diverse managed care reviewers who use that information to make reimbursement determinations. Current documentation methods for describing mental healthcare services are inadequate for this task.

The difficulty in extrapolating from the medical record what treatment is being implemented for a patient and why it was chosen is not a new concern. In 1969, Lawrence Weed commented that "at present no operational system exists that permits a medical teacher or member of an accrediting agency to take a patient's record . . . and assess whether current medical standards are being properly applied" (p. 122). Loosely structured and organized by diagnosis, the medical records of Dr. Weed's day were observed to be "simply static, pro forma repositories of medical observations and activities grouped in the meaningless order of source—whether doctor or nurse, laboratory or X-ray department" (p. vii). It was in reaction to this arcane and archaic method of collecting, organizing, and recording patient care data that the problem-oriented record was conceived and promulgated.

The "Weed system" introduced a documentation method that provided practitioners with a mechanism not only for recording the reasons (problems) for initiating patient care, but also, and more importantly, for graphically displaying the decision-making processes that determined the progress of that care. This system was designed to facilitate ready access to patient care data for meaningful treatment planning and concurrent case review as well as to expedite retrieval of data for retrospective research and education. The "patient problem list" and the "subjective-objective-assessment-plan" (SOAP) format were conceived as operational mechanisms for ensuring and expanding the usefulness of the patient record. The patient problem list was to be the dynamic reflection of the evolving thought process of the practitioner as well as a means of tracking the clinical progress of the patient.

When psychiatry seized the problem-oriented record and applied it to psychiatric inpatient care, the essential dynamism of the Weed system was either lost or abandoned. The "patient problems" currently found in psychiatric records appear to be no more than landings on which the treatment team rests rather than stairs that are used to document (communicate) the practitioners' evolving thought process and the patient's changing clinical course. Today's patient problem lists are cafeterias of unstandardized terms selected to meet the unwritten(!) requirement for a patient problem list. Psychiatric patient problems are typically adjectival descriptions (e.g., "attention-seeking behavior"), static conditions (e.g., "adoption issues"), critical judgments (e.g., "resistant to treatment"), theoretical constructs (e.g., "poor ego boundaries"), value statements (e.g., "poor peer choices"), anecdotal inferences (e.g., "demanding and dependent"), arbitrary conclusions (e.g., "poor impulse control"), or diagnoses (e.g., "dysthymia").

The above examples constituted a problem list in an actual hospital record. Such a list fails to document (communicate) why the patient (admitted with the diagnosis of Major Depression) needed treatment, why the various treatment services prescribed were necessary, and why an inpatient setting was required to implement them. A problem such as "adoption issues" contains no spectrum for change within its syntax, thereby paralyzing the practitioner's ability to communicate the patient's progress toward resolving the problem, and so conveys effectiveness of the treatment based on patient outcome.

Reviewers want to know how treatment decisions are made and what the clinical rationale is for each of them. An oft-heard comment from a reviewer is, "I may know what's going on with a patient, but I don't always know why." Again, this is because clinicians have not been educated about the value of articulating and documenting their own thought processes. The managed care review process inserts a number of questions between the time the practitioner establishes a diagnosis and the time he or she initiates the treatment. The reviewer wants to know why that treatment is necessary, why a particular treatment setting or frequency of service is required, and why alternative treatments are not considered appropriate. Lengthy problem lists and a multiplicity of treatment interventions do not adequately convey this information.

It is inevitable that before long *all* providers of mental healthcare services in *all* treatment settings (i.e., inpatient, partial hospitalization, residential treatment, and outpatient) will be required to document and communicate the process and quality of their care. As mentioned earlier, the Joint Commission is continually sharpening its focus and refining its parameters for measuring, assessing, and improving quality in mental healthcare in acute inpatient, partial hospital, residential, and outpatient treatment settings, as well as in integrated delivery systems (called healthcare networks). The collective assessment of the quality of each treatment modality (i.e., each potentially billable service) measures the overall quality of clinical care a patient receives.

In mental healthcare, several different professionals (e.g., psychiatrist, psychologist, or social worker) may perform the same service (e.g., individual psychotherapy). To measure, assess, and improve quality of mental healthcare, we conceptualize the written care plan (practitioner interventions) to be organized by treatment modality (e.g., individual psychotherapy) instead of by discipline or license (e.g., psychiatry, psychology, social work).

The treatment modalities utilized on a psychiatric inpatient service providing comprehensive multidisciplinary treatment might include, but are not limited to, the following:

- Individual psychotherapy
- Psychopharmacotherapy
- Electroconvulsive therapy
- Nursing
- Discharge planning (social services)
- Individual family therapy
- Multiple family therapy
- Group psychotherapy
- Occupational therapy
- Recreational therapy
- Creative arts therapy (e.g., psychodrama)
- Physical therapy
- Biofeedback therapy

- Substance abuse counseling
- Nutritional and dietary counseling
- Educational services

We are committed to the belief that an easy-to-use, operational treatment terminology utilizing clear, commonly understood, behavior-based language can communicate the measurable, objective process and quality of care to those individuals who need to know about it. Such a terminology does not require the mental health practitioner to forfeit or even necessarily compromise the appreciable, subjective quality of care—in all its subtlety and nuance—as currently understood and practiced. As consultants to practitioners, healthcare organizations, and patients who are appealing reimbursement denials from various managed care companies, we continue to be impressed that more than half of these denials result from inadequate communication of the reasons for treatment and the clinical rationale for the specific services requested. More often than not, the recommended care was clinically appropriate; however, the information exchange between the practitioner and the reviewer failed to communicate *why*. When practitioners can approach the review process as a request for clarity of thought, rather than a threat of nonpayment, they may well be able to respond artfully and more effectually to reviewers as colleagues and not as menacing strangers.

Chapter 4

Impairments and the Diagnosis

"What is the patient's diagnosis?"

Utilizing a common-language terminology of impairments *for describing patients with mental disorders prepares the provider to communicate the observable or reported reasons for treatment. The diagnosis describes the disorder the patient has; the impairments describe the manifestations of that diagnosis that will become the focus of treatment. Impairments also become the reimburser's tools for making payment determinations. The advantages of impairments as behavioral descriptors of patient dysfunctions are discussed, and a lexicon of impairments we have identified in patients seeking mental health treatment services is presented.*

The most commonly asked first question during an initial managed care review—for example, to obtain preauthorization for a hospitalization—is, "What is the patient's diagnosis?" We agree with Kiesler (1982) that additional information is necessary to describe a patient's current psychiatric condition and explain the clinical rationale for the proposed treatment. The treatment terminology we have devised to link the patient's diagnosis to the mental healthcare practitioner's planned interventions is the subject of this chapter.

Diagnosis is the conclusive evidence of the treater's ability to synthesize findings. After obtaining a thorough history, performing mental status and physical examinations, and reviewing all available ancillary data (e.g., laboratory tests, consultation reports, narrative accounts by observers), the treater calls on his or her skill, experience, and general fund of knowledge to formulate the nature of the condition—that is, the diagnosis. The practitioner then affixes the name of that condition to the patient. Establishing a diagnosis is intended to inform the practitioner how to proceed with treatment. More recently, diagnosis also has been employed to inform third-party payers and other external reviewers how much to reimburse for certain treatment services.

The Medicare Prospective Payment System (PPS) fixes the reimbursement for hospital medical-surgical treatment to particular diagnosis-related groups (DRGs). The DRGs are based on the arguable premise that a descriptive label of the disorder—a diagnosis—and the patient are synonymous or that the diagnosis so closely approximates the afflicted individual and the treatment that will be given that patient and diagnosis are interchangeable. Therefore, the costs to treat each are considered equivalent. Because the diagnostic nomenclature for describing psychiatric and chemical dependency patients does not by itself predict the treatment, psychiatry has maintained a DRG exemption from this mandated alliance between the diagnosis of a condition and the cost of treating a patient. As DSM-IV (American Psychiatric Association 1994) clearly cautions:

> A common misconception is that a classification of mental disorders classifies people, when actually what are being classified are disorders that people have. (p. xxii)

> To formulate an adequate treatment plan, the clinician will invariably require considerable additional information about the person being evaluated beyond that required to make a DSM-IV diagnosis. (p. xxv)

Psychiatric diagnoses are descriptors of complex mental states. Although certain diagnoses do in fact suggest specific medication treatment protocols, the DSM-IV nomenclature does not by itself predict the treatment setting or the treatment interventions necessary to care for the patient. In a study conducted 2 years after the publication of DSM-III-R (American Psychiatric Association 1987), it was found that one-third of psychiatrists continued to use DSM-III (American Psychiatric Association 1980) as their primary diagnostic reference (Zimmerman 1988). In 1994, DSM-IV was released to maintain a consistent terminology and coding system with the *International Classification of Diseases, 9th Revision, Clinical Modification* (ICD-9-CM) (World Health Organization 1980). Because patients can receive different diagnoses depending on the system that is used, reviewers encounter diagnoses that are now preceded by adjectives that are based on a specific classification system (e.g., the patient has a DSM-IV Dysthymic Disorder or a DSM-III-R Depressive Neurosis).

At a practical level, clinicians are occasionally confronted with the problem of explaining diagnostic changes to outside reviewers. Reviewers get frustrated when they see multiple psychiatric diagnoses over time for the same patient. Trying to explain that a previous physician was using a different nomenclature does not appease them. At the other end of the spectrum, reviewers are also baffled when the entire patient population on a psychiatric unit carries the same diagnosis of "major depression." These changing definitions of pathological conditions can confound the review process and argue for a consistent and descriptive treatment terminology that can be used to document the reasons (objectively manifest or subjectively reported) why a patient needs care.

This is not an original idea. The psychiatric nursing profession has already conceptualized a compendium of treatment descriptors for its own use. At the 1981 American Nursing Association Congress on Nursing Practice, the profession staked its claim to diagnose and treat selected "health problems" using behaviorally referenced "nursing diagnoses" that "objectify perceived difficulties or needs by naming them as a basis for understanding and taking action to resolve the concerns" (Kim et al. 1984, p. 26). These descriptors, endorsed by the North American Nursing Diagnosis Association (NANDA), represented the first organized effort to catalog patient behaviors systematically and link them to treatment intervention and outcome.

NANDA diagnoses structure the nursing care plan, and their concreteness and objectivity are valuable aids for monitoring and evaluating patient progress. In those psychiatric facilities where the written treatment plan is the responsibility of nursing professionals, these nursing diagnoses often become a generic treatment documentation language of their own. By definition and design, however, these terms are limited to the scope of the discipline. Some NANDA nursing diagnoses (e.g., "ineffective individual coping" and "alterations in thought process") are not serviceable to other mental health disciplines and either are precariously close to value judgments or represent inferential conclusions about static patient states or traits.

A number of exhaustive and comprehensive attempts have been made to systematize or codify a standard set of patient problems. However, the difficulty we found in a review of a number of dictionaries of psychiatric patient problems (e.g., Longabaugh et al. 1983; Meldman et al. 1976; Problem-Oriented Medical Record Project 1978) and for treatment planning (Angle et al. 1977; Ryback et al. 1981) is that they all define *problem* with numerous parameters and overly broad guidelines. The resulting voluminous lists of terms only variably convince a reviewer why a patient needs particular services and why a specific treatment setting is required to provide them.

Patient problem lists also do not systematically capture a patient's particular strengths and the comorbid conditions that may have an impact on the anticipated patient outcome for particular treatments. An articulate, motivated, responsible, and introspective patient may reach the goals of treatment in less time and at less expense than an individual who does not possess these particular strengths. On the other hand, an adolescent patient hospitalized for an acute schizophrenic episode who also has a learning disability, a major educational deficit, and lives with parents who are active substance abusers may require more treatment efforts (at additional expense) than would be necessary to treat the schizophrenic episode without these additional comorbid conditions.

Based on these observed shortcomings of current nosologies and organizational formats for documenting the treatment of psychiatric patients, we have developed a common-language terminology for documenting mental healthcare. This terminology has the following features:

1. Communicates the reasons for, and notarizes the appropriateness of, treatment
2. Identifies the comorbid conditions and captures all adverse occurrences that may impact the course (and outcome) of treatment
3. Is demonstrably behavioral, prompting practitioners to document (and communicate) objectified, behavioral progress toward patient objectives
4. Includes all the mental health issues identified in DSM-IV and psychiatric NANDA diagnoses
5. Cogently, succinctly, and humanistically describes patient difficulties, from the initial visit (or preadmission screening) to the termination of treatment and follow-up
6. Is serviceable to all practitioners, regardless of their theoretical or clinical orientation
7. Coordinates a diversity of treatment modalities toward consensually agreed-on patient dysfunctions and their remediation
8. Can be easily learned and understood by individuals in all mental health disciplines and health professionals in other disciplines
9. Is compatible with the biological, psychological, behavioral, and family and social system models that currently contribute to the understanding and treatment of psychiatric disorders

We recommend that the behavioral dysfunctions for which patients appropriately seek and require mental health services primarily—and the identified conditions that may impact their treatment secondarily—be identified as patient "impairments." *Impairment* describes a worsened, lessened, weakened, damaged, or reduced ability to function and, in turn, anticipates a potential for repair, improvement, enhancement, and strengthening. The impairments identified in this book were selected for their power to signal the appropriateness for treatment and frame the documentation and communication of not only the treatment plan but also the patient's response to treatment interventions.

Impairments are the reasons why a patient requires treatment. They are not the reasons for the presence of the disorder, nor are they the disorder itself. Rather, they are observable, objectifiable manifestations that necessitate and justify care.

Impairments can be regarded as the actional expressions of the DSM-IV diagnoses, their psychodynamic explanations (e.g., "poor ego boundaries"), and their neurobiological origins (e.g., serotonin deficiency). Impairments are "behavioral windows" into the aberrant biochemical phenomena and psychological variations of existence that are the etiology of psychiatric disorders. The treatment interventions prescribed for impairments are chosen for their ability to "repair" the disordered behaviors manifestly by correcting (ultimately) these biological dysregulations and experiential aberrations.

Comprehensive assessment of the patient's operational world (internal and external) is necessary for restoration and maintenance of biopsychosocial completeness (Marmor 1982). This "holistic" approach is the basis for the "concentric sphere" paradigm we employ when describing the patient. Each sphere locates a number of potential impairments that mental healthcare practitioners may identify in patients whom they are assessing for treatment (see Figure 4–1).

Impairments may be located in both the patient's subjectively experienced "private" world and the objectively measured "public" or actional world. In our model, the patient's *biopsychology* is represented at the center, circumscribed by an anatomic skin boundary (which metaphorically encloses the patient's internal world or inner reality as well). Spheres

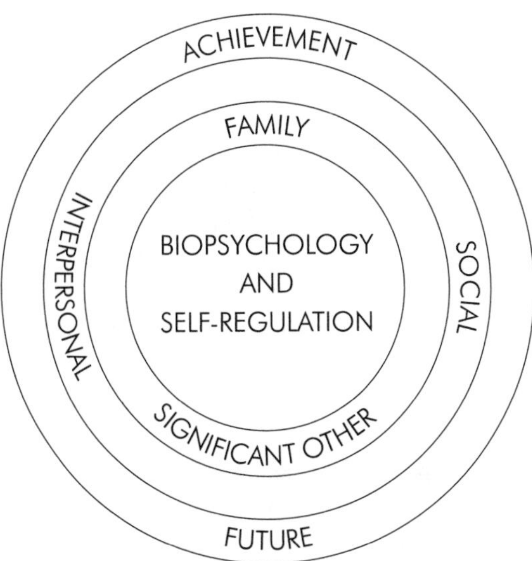

Figure 4–1. The patient's operational world.

"outside" this boundary (but still "within" the patient's larger world) include the proximate and critically influential sphere of the *family/significant other* and the larger, developmentally postponed sphere of the *social/interpersonal*. Outermost is the sphere of the *future/achievement*. The impairments that are assigned to each of these spheres are now presented. (See Appendix A for the impairment definitions.)

Biopsychology Impairments

The integrative concept of biopsychology updates a traditional demarcation between body (biology) and mind (psychology). The separation of "psyche" and "soma" is no longer metapsychologically explanatory or neurophysiologically valid. With respect to the psychoses, for example, it is now apparent that they may be either "psycho-somatic" or "somatopsychic" conditions (Grotstein et al. 1987). A psychosomatic alteration of the central nervous system following perceived catastrophic events may so alter the neurological mind that a secondary psychosomatic defect in mental processing is set in motion. The somatopsychic psychosis is an inherited defective neurological organization that is so fragile and hypersensitive to the stimuli of emotional experience that a disorganization of the central nervous system is too easily evoked. The consequence is a secondary psychic disorganization.

Biological givens (heredity) and experiential aberrations (environment) are conciliatorily understood in this model as reciprocal influences that are interdependent and interfacilitating. The impairments assigned to the sphere of biopsychology are the behavioral derivatives of (and windows to) neurophysiological, anatomical, biochemical, and experiential aberrations and their interplay. Hallucinations, for example, may be "explained" as a symptom of schizophrenia, which in itself is explained by neurobiological aberrations that lead to a faulty processing of experiential data, making "non-sense" out of "sense-ory" input from the real world (Flannery and Taylor 1981; Heilbrunn 1979; Meyersburg and Post 1979; Taylor 1985). To the outside reviewer, a diagnosis of schizophrenia implies a chronic, progressive disease. In our model, we do not include schizophrenia as an impairment because it does not communicate to a reviewer why a particular type of treatment is needed at a given point in time. That the patient has the impairment of Hallucinations that, for example, are invoking thoughts of suicide is more to the point.

Impairments in the biopsychology sphere include behaviors that mediate between the patient's internal world and external reality to regulate, preserve, and restore psychological (and/or biological) homeostasis. Disorders of self-regulation are the actional (and at times desperate) efforts of the patient to maintain or restore psychological equilibrium in the face of painfully experienced tension states ranging from fleeting signal anxiety to profound dread, panic, and threats of psychological catastrophe. These tension states may spontaneously arise from within (neurophysiological dysregulation) or may be prompted by external stressors (environmental overload or deprivation). In either case, they impinge on and threaten to harm the patient.

For example, obsessive-compulsive disorder was formerly understood only as a neurotic resolution of the anal phase of development and sadistic fantasies directed toward the object. Empirical psychobiological psychiatry now tells us that the "obsessive-compulsive neurosis" may also be a screen to defend against biological affective disorders, principally depressive or panic disorders (Behar et al. 1984; Elkins et al. 1980; Hoover and Insel 1984). The function of the obsessive-compulsive symptoms—and of phobias for that matter—is to circumscribe the area of biochemical defect and take active, fantasied measures (symptoms) to demarcate it and avoid it. Obsessive-compulsive disorder and other related disorders, therefore, may now be best treated with the combination of medication and psychotherapy. Such behaviors as bulimia and chemical dependence are also understood in this model as self-regulatory efforts "to feel good again" through the desperate behaviors of purging and liver cell destruction. When examined from this point of view, suicide is a desperate act contemplated or carried out to regulate oneself against such intolerable affect states.

The impairments we have defined as belonging to the sphere of biopsychology are listed in Table 4–1.

Family/Significant Other Impairments

Impairments in the patient's ability to relate to others are often the first ones to signal the patient's appropriate need for mental health services. Although it is axiomatic that the role of the immediate family and significant other may be critical and even explanatory for the pathogenesis of patient dysfunctions, such difficulties may not by themselves justify more intensive treatment settings. Impairments in the family/significant other sphere are identified whenever such family interventions are able to facilitate whatever therapeutic progress is realistic or possible in a given

Table 4–1. Impairments in the biopsychology sphere

Alexithymia	Medical Risk Factor
Altered Sleep	Mood Lability
Anxiety	Motor Hyperactivity
Compulsions	Obsessions
Concomitant Medical Condition	Pathological Grief
Decreased Concentration	Pathological Guilt
Delusions (Nonparanoid)	Phobia
Delusions (Paranoid)	Promiscuity
Dissociative State	Psychomotor Retardation
Dysphoric Mood	Psychotic Thought/Behavior
Eating Disorder	Self-Esteem Deficiency
Encopresis	Self-Mutilation
Enuresis	Somatization
Externalization and Blame	Stealing
Fire Setting	Substance Abuse
Gender Dysphoria	Suicidal Thought/Behavior
Hallucinations	Uncontrolled Buying
Learning Disability	Uncontrolled Gambling
Manic Thought/Behavior	

clinical situation. Specific field resistances to patient progress may be reduced through selective family interventions (S. L. Brown 1980). Those interventions may occur occasionally, only once, or fairly often in the course of therapy with a designated patient. Treatment for a patient's biopsychology impairments may be facilitated by treating the patient's impairments in the family/significant other sphere as well.

The impairments we have identified in the sphere of family/significant other are listed in Table 4–2.

Table 4–2. Impairments in the family/significant other sphere

Emotional Abuse Perpetrator	Physical Abuse Perpetrator
Emotional Abuse Victim	Physical Abuse Victim
Family Dysfunction	Sexual Trauma Perpetrator
Marital/Relationship Dysfunction	Sexual Trauma Victim
Marital/Relationship Dysfunction With Substance Abuse	Running Away

Social/Interpersonal Impairments

Impairments in the social/interpersonal sphere document the patient's chaotic, confusing, unmanageable, or frankly overwhelming external world. This is a world characterized by destructive, dangerous relationships or behaviors that ultimately affect the patient and others. The treatment plan must respond to these difficulties to provide a consistent and durable environment in which the patient can improve overall functioning. It may be critical to the survival of the treatment (and the patient) for the practitioner to intervene in destructive relationships and repair and facilitate healthy, supportive ones while treating the patient's biopsychology impairments. Impairments in the social/interpersonal sphere, such as Oppositionalism or Social Withdrawal, will continue to compromise patient functioning in his or her world despite optimal treatment of, for example, the impairments of Hyperactivity or Psychotic Thought/Behavior. The social/interpersonal impairments can be the comorbid conditions that ultimately determine the success or failure of treatment.

Impairments we have identified in the social/interpersonal sphere are listed in Table 4–3.

Future/Achievement Impairments

In addition to the restoration of biopsychosocial completeness referenced earlier, there is a restoration of temporal completeness that we offer to our patients. We not only pay attention to what *was* (both constitutionally and experientially) and what *is* (behaviorally and biochemically), but we also address the treatable difficulties that obstruct or paralyze the patients' ability to plan and propel themselves into the future—for what *will be.* This is the sphere in which plans for the future, ambition for setting new

Table 4–3. Impairments in the social/interpersonal sphere

Assaultiveness	Sexual Performance Dysfunction
Egocentricity	Sexual Object Choice Dysfunction
Homicidal Thought/Behavior	Social Withdrawal
Lying	Tantrums
Manipulativeness	Uncommunicativeness
Oppositionalism	

Table 4–4. Impairments in the future/achievement sphere

Educational Performance Deficit	Medical Treatment Noncompliance
Inadequate Healthcare Skills	School Avoidance
Inadequate Self-Maintenance Skills	Truancy

goals, and the hope for tomorrow have atrophied, become derailed, or been forfeited regardless of the cause.

Impairments we have identified in the sphere of future/achievement are listed in Table 4–4.

Conclusion

It either has or will become obvious to the reader that the categorization of the impairments in the concentric sphere paradigm is somewhat arbitrary. The lists of impairments for each sphere may not be definitively complete or exhaustive. These obvious shortcomings notwithstanding, we have found this model useful for the comprehensive identification of the patient's impairments that mental healthcare practitioners may address in their treatment plan. How we employ the impairment language to structure and organize the communication and documentation of all phases of patient care—from the initial intake assessment to the termination of treatment—is the subject of the remaining chapters in this book.

Chapter 5

Impairments and the Justification for Treatment

"Please tell me about the patient."

In this chapter, we demonstrate the utility of the impairments for communicating why a patient requires mental health services. We present 12 patient vignettes and detail the rationale for identifying the specific impairments for each patient.

The assessment of patients by systematically examining the "concentric spheres" of their internal and external operational worlds (see Chapter 4) encourages the identification of multiple impairments. When learning the impairment terminology, the practitioner may wish first to compile an "impairment inventory." This inventory uses the impairment terminology to summarize all the cognitive, affective, and behavioral disturbances manifested by the patient during the initial assessment. The impairment inventory then becomes a part of the assessment. The next step is to select from the inventory those impairments that 1) most convincingly describe why the patient needs treatment now and 2) will be the focus of the practitioner's treatment interventions. The selection criteria presented here, like the impairment inventory, are easily learned and soon become "automatic" functions. For the balance of this chapter, we refer to the impairments selected for treatment as the *patient impairment list*. This selection process is, of course, a subjective determination that evidences the practitioner's skill both to assess *and* to treat. This process provides valuable practitioner performance data that are now preserved in the patient impairment list.

To avoid the creation of a "stuffed" patient impairment list that names every problem, potential or real, treatable or not treatable, we caution the practitioner to select only those impairments targeted for "repair" or treatment at a particular level of care. In our experience, a lengthy, or stuffed, list of treatment concerns does a disservice both to the patient and to the practitioner by blurring the specific reasons for which treatment is recommended. A large number of potential or, in some cases, unresolvable impairments may not justify treatment at all. In addition, just one critically severe impairment *may* require, and be appropriately treated at, the most service-intensive level of care.

To this end, the practitioner selects the impairments that will be the focus of treatment based on the following criteria:

1. The impairment describes patient behaviors and/or patient statements that can be objectified and quantified.
2. The impairment will be actively addressed in the treatment plan.
3. The impairment is reasonably anticipated to improve with treatment.

4. The impairment is not inconsistent with the DSM-IV (American Psychiatric Association 1994) criteria for the patient's diagnosis.
5. The patient's impairment list, when completed, reflects examination of all spheres of the patient's world.
6. An impairment may (secondarily) impact the treatment of another (primary) impairment.

We recommend that the impairments be hierarchically listed, with the biopsychology impairments listed first. The impairment language is designed to communicate succinctly and accurately the clinical necessity for mental healthcare services. A subgroup of impairments has the potential to become more severe than others and can justify more intensive treatment services (e.g., inpatient hospitalization). More will be said about rating the severity of the impairments in Chapter 6.

In our experience with managed care reviewers, the impairments provide a convenient outline to respond expeditiously to the often first-stated, and at times disquietingly vague, request, "Please tell me about the patient." Our response to this opening request is to state the patient's age, race, marital status, sex, and occupation and then proceed directly to the reasons why the patient is seeking treatment. We let the reviewer know (either by telephone or written communication) that we have devised an impairment list and explain that it is a summary of the issues to be addressed in the treatment plan. We indicate that we would like to refer to this list when discussing the patient throughout the course of treatment.

To those reviewers who choose to follow the traditional medical-surgical model by requesting the patient's diagnosis, we do provide the initial DSM-IV diagnosis and then specify either the principal diagnosis or the reason for the visit. We try to avoid offering Axis II diagnoses when possible for several reasons:

1. There is considerable confusion surrounding these diagnoses, which describe "persistent personality traits," and there is a lack of well-established validation of their diagnostic criteria and outcome with or without treatment (Vaillant and Perry 1985).
2. "The diagnostic categories, criteria, and textual descriptions are meant to be employed by individuals with appropriate clinical training and experience in diagnosis" (American Psychiatric Association 1994, p. xxiii).
3. Some review organizations, without clear research-based criteria on which to rely, exclude personality disorders from mental health benefits.

4. A growing body of literature is now reporting a temporal link between the major psychiatric disorders and the personality disorders (Othmer and Othmer 1989).

Offering the diagnosis of a personality disorder, unfortunately, suggests to some reviewers a chronic clinical condition and thus impedes the task at hand—which is to communicate (and document) why the patient needs treatment and why he or she needs it *now*.

The DSM-IV V codes and "Other Conditions That May Be a Focus of Clinical Attention" pose similar difficulties, and we avoid them as well. Their respective definitions either exclude or de-emphasize the presence of a treatable mental disorder, and this serves only to call into question why the patient requires *mental* healthcare services. As noted, we have encountered some external review organizations that have identified personality disorders and V codes as either red flags for more in-depth review or outright exclusion criteria for reimbursement. The offering of such "supplemental" diagnostic information can hamper the practitioner's communication of the clinical necessity for treatment.

Case Histories

We present here 12 patient vignettes, selected to exemplify some of the more common clinical presentations mental health practitioners may frequently encounter. The first five vignettes demonstrate the use of the impairment list for patients requiring acute inpatient care. The second five illustrate the use of the impairment list for patients receiving outpatient services. The last two vignettes demonstrate the utility of the impairment list for describing chronic conditions with acute exacerbations that necessitate treatment.

The impairment list that we developed for each patient is provided, along with the DSM-IV Axis I and Axis II diagnoses. The rationale for the selection of the particular impairments in each list is detailed where necessary. We wish to reiterate that the impairment terminology is not designed to compete or conflict with DSM-IV nomenclature, which does not classify patients but rather classifies "disorders that people have" (American Psychiatric Association 1994, p. xxii). Impairment terminology bridges the gap between the diagnosis and the treatment interventions. Impairments structure the documentation of mental healthcare services and the communication of a clear rationale as to why those services are necessary.

We ask that special attention be given to the first two vignettes—Melanie W. and Bob D.—because these two cases will be used as clinical examples throughout the remainder of the book to demonstrate the utility of the impairments for determining severity ratings, creating goals and patient objectives, and identifying treatment interventions. The reader is again reminded that this impairment terminology is neither definitive nor exhaustive; "impairments" other than those we have identified in Chapter 4 may be "created" by practitioners and should be included for their own use. What is essential is that any new term selected be demonstrably *behavioral* and contain behavioral manifestations with realistic potential for quantifiable improvement. The reasons for this are explained in the subsequent chapters.

Case 1: Melanie W.

History

Melanie W., a 17-year-old high school student with juvenile-type diabetes mellitus, was referred for psychiatric hospitalization from a hospital facility specializing in chronic medical disease. Prior to her medical hospital admission, Melanie had been refusing to self-administer her insulin regularly, was frequently disregarding her diabetic diet, and, when angry or depressed, would "regulate" her mood by readjusting her insulin dose to precipitate severe hypo- or hyperglycemic episodes.

She presented to the emergency room as a brittle, juvenile-onset–type diabetic whose blood glucose was measured at 415 mg/100 ml. Historically, Melanie's blood glucose was very difficult to control, and she had been hospitalized more than 20 times for severe hyperglycemic episodes. When her condition was sufficiently stabilized in the hospital for her to adjust her twice daily insulin doses on a fixed schedule based on her blood glucose (which she tested herself in the morning and late afternoon), Melanie was referred for psychiatric evaluation. She stated that she could not make the commitment to follow this regimen on her own responsibly.

Melanie readily acknowledged her intent to deviate from the recommended insulin doses despite the potentially life-threatening consequences. She reported feeling "different from other kids" ever since she knew she had the disease and stated she did not care if she died early. She also admitted that she had no intention of curtailing intake of foods with high sugar content. Melanie was very knowledgeable about her diabetes, its management, and its clinical course, but she was unwilling to tailor her lifestyle to meet the demands of the illness.

Melanie's attendance at school had been erratic, and her educational performance had been very poor. The local school board was threatening legal action against the parents for tolerating, if not outrightly encouraging, Melanie's habitual truancy. Melanie's mother admitted that she was unable to get Melanie to go to school and, in fact, stated it was easier for her to have Melanie at home to help take care of Melanie's 8-month-old brother. Melanie saw no reason to attend school and had no future goals for herself, although she thought she might get married and have children someday.

Melanie's family life was very chaotic. She was the eldest of six children. Her father worked 6 days a week, 10–12 hours a day, and he unabashedly acknowledged that he was "not involved in the family" other than to complain about his wife's ineffectiveness with the children, the problems with which he felt his children burdened him, and the long hours of work necessary to support the family. Melanie's mother was quick to disclose that she was "quite disorganized" and was aware of her ineffectiveness in carrying out household responsibilities and in being a parent. Family chores were not defined, and the household ran on a crisis model. Although all eight family members lived in a three-bedroom home, Melanie had her own bedroom. The parents reported that this was due to Melanie's inability to get along with her siblings. Melanie, however, experienced this as further evidence that she was the "sick one" who needed to be isolated from the rest of the family. This isolation, in turn, reinforced her reclusiveness.

Clinical Presentation

Melanie presented as a moderately overweight high school student who was poorly groomed, unkempt, sullen, and slow to respond. Speech was visibly an effort for her, and she strained to find words, which she uttered just above a whisper. She was alert and coherent, although her use of language was somewhat childish.

She reported experiencing life as hopeless and seemed blandly indifferent to the life-threatening consequences of her intentional mismanagement of her diabetes. She looked puzzled when it was suggested that she might be angry about the severe imposition and limitations the diabetes exerted on her life. She said she never experienced anger and, in fact, stated that she did not think she really knew what anger was. She denied any active suicidal intent, while at the same time acknowledging the seriousness and potential lethality of her behavior. There was no evidence of active psychosis or any organic impairment.

Assessment

Although Melanie denied active suicidal ideation, the impairment of Suicidal Thought/Behavior was chosen because her behavior was indeed life threatening, and Melanie would require close supervision to ensure her safety. Melanie's depression manifested behaviorally with a visible and verbalized Dysphoric Mood. Her blatant refusal to manage her Concomitant Medical Condition—the diabetes—would require close medical supervision and psychotherapy. Her poor grooming, poor hygiene, and indifference to her diabetic management were three aspects of her Inadequate Healthcare Skills that would require monitoring, education, and repair. The Family Dysfunction and Truancy were self-evident. Melanie was admitted to an inpatient psychiatric unit with a diagnosis of Major Depressive Disorder (DSM-IV).

Patient: Melanie W.

Diagnosis:

Axis I: Major Depressive Disorder, Single Episode, Severe, Without Psychotic Features (296.23)

Axis II: None

Impairments:

1. **Suicidal Thought/Behavior**
2. **Dysphoric Mood**
3. **Concomitant Medical Condition (juvenile-type diabetes mellitus)**
4. **Inadequate Healthcare Skills**
5. **Family Dysfunction**
6. **Truancy**

* *Note to the reader: Major Depression (DSM-III-R) (American Psychiatric Association 1987)—or Major Depressive Disorder (DSM-IV)—is a frequently used diagnosis for psychiatric inpatients. When we reviewed a year's admissions to a 95-bed private psychiatric hospital (where Melanie was treated), we found that more than 75% of the patients were admitted and discharged with that diagnosis. Yet, the impairment profiles we had for these patients demonstrated a very diverse range of treatment concerns. Melanie's impairment profile, although containing more impairments than most of the patient records we reviewed, is very patient specific. Inadequate Healthcare Skills is used, rather than Medication Treatment Noncompliance, because Melanie's poor self-care went beyond her noncompliance. The single "umbrella" of Inadequate Healthcare Skills was chosen to capture both the mismanagement of her diabetes and her poor hygiene and self-care.*

Case 2: Bob D.

History

Bob, a 23-year-old, was brought to a medical emergency room by his parents who were called by two of Bob's friends to tell them Bob had been "talking all night about performing, stating that he was a messenger from God." The friends reported that Bob was variously claiming that he could "move buildings and rearrange the city streets with his 'special powers'" and that he had the authority to "seize in the name of the Lord" a commercial warehouse to "convert it to a child's theme park." The friends also added, "One minute Bob said he was the 'God of Gods,' and the next minute he would call himself a 'chief of city planning chiefs.'" The parents picked Bob up and brought him to the emergency room for evaluation.

Bob's mother reported that Bob had been terminated recently from his job because of tardiness, absenteeism, and argumentativeness and that he had been married for just over a year. Bob had previously lived at home after completing high school and 1 year at a junior college. He had occasionally worked as an auto mechanic's assistant, but the parents confided that he had "never found a place to work where he was happy." Bob and his wife had continued to be largely dependent on his family for financial support. Bob's wife was also concerned about Bob's drinking "at least four to six beers a day" and his association with "people who didn't do much of anything but drink and 'hang out.'" Whenever attempts had been made by the family to discuss some of these behaviors with Bob, he became very angry, screamed obscenities, shook his fists in the air, and would often storm out of the house and occasionally be gone for 1 or 2 days at a time. Any moderate impasse provoked such reactions.

Clinical Presentation

In the emergency room, Bob presented as a handsome, muscular, adult male, visibly agitated and obviously preoccupied. He could engage in the interview for only a minute or so before repeating very emphatically that he was God's chosen messenger and had been given the mission to save the children of the city by redesigning the streets and buildings. He smelled of alcohol, his speech was slurred, and he was moderately ataxic. He talked exuberantly about plans to perform "God's miracles" for "curing the sick and dying" and to "install more playgrounds and parks for children." He did not appear to be experiencing any hallucinations. There was no suicidal or homicidal ideation. He knew the month and the year but not the date or day of the week. He became argumentative on further questioning and stormed out of the room when psychiatric hospitalization was suggested. His parents were able to convince him, however, to sign himself in voluntarily.

Assessment

Although Bob is obviously both delusional and psychotic, it is unnecessary to include both Delusions (Nonparanoid) and Psychotic Thought/Behavior in the profile. The most accurate descriptor in this case is Delusions (Nonparanoid). The selection of the impairment of Substance Abuse (Alcohol) is straightforward enough. Because of Bob's inability to manage the demands of full-time employment, the volatility and eruptive behavior he displayed when anyone tried to discuss particularly sensitive issues with him, and his immature reactions (e.g., kicking and throwing things, stomping off yelling) when he would not get his way or always be the one who was right in any discussion, the impairment of Tantrums was included. Although this is not an impairment that in itself necessitates hospitalization,the presence of Bob's Tantrums could no doubt complicate his treatment. This comorbid condition would require its own specialized therapeutic interventions while Bob was in the acute treatment setting.

Patient: Bob D.

Diagnosis:

Axis I: Psychotic Disorder Not Otherwise Specified (298.9); Alcohol Intoxication (303.00)
Axis II: None

Impairments:

1. **Delusions (Nonparanoid)**
2. **Substance Abuse (Alcohol)**
3. **Tantrums**

Case 3: Sarah C.

History

Sarah, a 13-year-old, was admitted to the hospital because of her relentless carving on her arms and legs with kitchen tools and jackknives. Words, names of friends, and religious symbols were "tattooed" in scabs and scars on her forearms and thighs. She was also abusing alcohol daily and had been showing sudden changes in mood from vegetative social withdrawal to agitated, angry contrariness. These mood swings were increasing in frequency over the last half year. Sarah reported that she in fact enjoyed carving on herself, loved drinking alcohol, did not want to attend school, and hated her stepfather. The only thing she liked about "him and his rules" was the "fun in breaking them." She stated that she drank because it felt good and that she would stop "if my mother asked me to, but she never has."

Sarah's mother presented as a very anxious, visibly overwhelmed woman who appeared frightened by her daughter. Sarah's mother herself had had a long history of depression, requiring numerous hospitalizations, and of being "too sensitive to medication to take any."

Sarah's biological father had died when Sarah was 11 years old; however, he and Sarah's mother had divorced when Sarah was 2. Sarah had continued to remain very close to her biological father, visiting him quite often until his death. Her mother had married Sarah's stepfather when Sarah was 6. Sarah now lived with her mother, maternal grandmother, and stepfather. Her stepfather was a law enforcement officer and presented as gruff and authoritarian, with a narrow yet pragmatic view of the world. He and Sarah were obviously engaged in a power struggle, with her mother helplessly caught in the middle.

Clinical Presentation

Sarah presented as an unkempt, young Caucasian adolescent who looked several years older than her stated age. She was dressed in a "heavy metal" style—black chunky clothing, black ripped nylons, heavy jewelry—with one side of her head shaved. The baldness was covered by combing her very long hair across from the other side.

Sarah argued with any observation made about her, at times even contradicting her own statements made only minutes earlier. Simple requests (e.g., physical examination, routine blood testing) were met with complaints, arguments, or frank refusal. She denied being actively suicidal, although she drank to the point of intoxication and carved on herself almost daily. No hallucinations, delusions, or organic impairments were evidenced.

At the end of the assessment, her mother also revealed that Sarah and her stepsister were dependents of the court because of parental neglect. The family had been investigated for the parents' repeated failure to register the children in school, and the physical condition of the home was found to be unsafe and unsanitary.

Assessment

This is a severe and difficult case, with a number of acute problems identified in her impairment list justifying intensive, well-supervised treatment interventions. The criticalness of the Self-Mutilation and Substance Abuse (Alcohol) is self-evident. A biological contribution to the Mood Lability would need to be considered, especially in light of the family history of affective disorder. Sarah's Oppositionalism would need to be addressed as a specific treatment concern to facilitate repair of the more critical and severe impairments. The lack of family support and the absence of family structure (i.e., Family Dysfunction) made recidivism a major risk. The effects of the parental neglect on Sarah and her reactions to public investigation and being in legal custody of the court would also require exploration and understanding.

Patient: Sarah C.

Diagnosis:

Axis I: Cyclothymic Disorder (301.13); rule out Bipolar I Disorder (296.7)
Axis II: Borderline Personality Disorder (301.83)

Impairments:

1. **Self-Mutilation**
2. **Mood Lability**
3. **Substance Abuse (Alcohol)**
4. **Oppositionalism**
5. **Family Dysfunction**
6. **Physical Abuse Victim**

✻ *Note to the reader: We believe this (also rather long) impairment list clearly conveys the tangible issues that the treatment team would be addressing while Sarah was in the hospital. Although the last three impairments are customarily treated in outpatient settings, their presence in this case will impact the treatment of the first three impairments, and they are therefore included in the impairment list. The last impairment, Physical Abuse Victim, includes—by definition—the suffering from neglect as well. Hence, it is not necessary to include Emotional Abuse Victim in this list.*

Case 4: George G.

History

George, a 19-year-old single high school graduate, was brought into treatment by his stepmother and father, who had become concerned about his increasing isolation from the family and few friends he had made while still in school. The parents also had noticed a deterioration in his personal hygiene over the last 6–8 months.

George had always verbalized his preference to remain at home and "help out the family." He never developed any outside interests and avoided any discussion with his family about emancipating himself or living on his own. George's parents had hoped he would "grow out of this" and were now concerned that he had not. George reported that he was frightened of people his own age, believing they would hurt him physically or make fun of him. He preferred the company of children 10 or more years his junior because "I can take care of them, and they like the same things I do."

He reported that life at home with his stepmother was without strife and that he was glad she and his father let him spend much of the day in his room daydreaming. George had disclosed to his stepmother that he had been physically abused by his biological mother and stepfather after his natural parents divorced when he was 3. When he was 8, George came to live with his biological father, who had remarried. George explained, "My real mother wanted me out of the house, and I wanted to live with my real father."

He reported that he felt safe in his new home but had never come to feel safe outside of it. School was always frightening for him. He had only a few acquaintances and never dated. After eight sessions of outpatient individual psychotherapy, George's condition was continuing to deteriorate.

Clinical Presentation

George presented as a timid, suspicious, tense, stiffly postured, less-than-tidy, thin, young adult male who was visibly uncomfortable in the interview. He spoke clearly but tersely and in a monotone. He reported feeling very lonely at times and remarked that he was even frightened by the interview. He denied any suicidal or homicidal ideation. He verbalized peculiar vague ideas regarding people and their motives—"People only talk to you if they want to get something out of you or hurt you."

Despite his severe social isolation and very poor interpersonal skills, George verbalized some rather grandiose expectations for himself in life—"I don't have to work or go to school; my parents will always be there." He denied experiencing anything that no one else did, and there were no bizarre or paranoid beliefs in evidence. He was oriented to time, place, and person. His immediate, recent, and remote memory were intact. He denied using alcohol or other drugs of abuse. His insights were very limited; his judgment was immature and poor.

Assessment

This case illustrates particularly well the effectiveness of the impairments for articulating a rationale for treatment. George's clinical presentation of a subchronic schizophrenic disorder does not by itself justify an "acute" diagnosis. The diagnosis, of course, describes only the category of disorders into which George's symptoms best fit. Yet, at the same time, he is clearly experiencing severe and compromising difficulties that warrant treatment intervention.

Whether the label for George's disorder is a schizophrenia (undifferentiated type or paranoid type) or a schizoaffective disorder is of less concern to an outside reviewer than the reasons why treatment is being recommended now. Not only did George fail to respond to outpatient treatment, but his impairments of Delusions (Paranoid), Psychotic Thought/Behavior, and Social Withdrawal were sufficiently disabling to warrant a more intensive level of care. Inadequate Healthcare Skills, Family Dysfunction, and Physical Abuse Victim would also require attention in the treatment, although by themselves these impairments are usually treated in outpatient settings.

Patient: George G.

Diagnosis:

Axis I: Schizophrenia, Undifferentiated Type, Episodic With Prominent Negative Symptoms (295.90)
Axis II: Schizotypal Personality Disorder (301.22)

Impairments:

1. **Delusions (Paranoid)**
2. **Psychotic Thought/Behavior**
3. **Social Withdrawal**
4. **Inadequate Healthcare Skills**
5. **Family Dysfunction**
6. **Physical Abuse Victim**

Case 5: David C.

History

David, a 16-year-old high school student, was brought in for psychiatric evaluation by his mother, who had become frightened by her son's violent behaviors. David and his mother were interviewed conjointly first, then David was examined individually. His mother reported feeling terrified by David's volatile and explosive verbal assaults in response to what she regarded as benign, noninvasive questions or requests (e.g., help with a household chore). Although destruction of household property (doors, furniture, glassware) was not uncommon, there had been no physical altercations between David and his mother. David reported feeling very guilty after each fight—"after I had a couple of hours to cool down"—and although he felt his mother was too intrusive and demanding, he stated he knew that she was doing the best she could.

David never knew his father. David reported being frequently in fights in and after school and openly admitted that he often hurt those he fought. He typically believed it was "they" who started any altercation (verbal or physical), and it was up to him to "finish it—physically." On one occasion, he got into a fight with a gas station attendant whom he had never met before.

David knew that he had seriously injured the man but had left before police arrived. He only remembered being "flooded with anger" and feeling completely out of control. David also reported difficulty keeping any part-time jobs because of his volatility. He often felt that "adults are always trying to take advantage of me." David verbalized feeling very depressed about himself, feeling that he was a "screwup and would probably only end up being a bum." He did not believe he could be a success at anything. He thought a great deal about dying but denied any active suicidal ideation or plan. He had not been attending school and was thinking about dropping out altogether. Interestingly, David had joined a 12-step program and reported being free of drugs and alcohol for the last 8 months.

Clinical Presentation

David presented as a vigorous, handsome, muscular, stern-looking, and tensely postured adolescent who appeared "on the alert," suspicious, and ready to defend himself physically. His speech was fluent and coherent. His affect was broodingly serious, and he was easily angered. He never smiled. David was very self-deprecating and self-condemning, and he doubted that anyone or anything could be of help to him. He posited that dying was one way to escape the pain of living but denied any specific plan. No overt psychotic thinking or organic impairment was in evidence.

Assessment

This complicated case is included to exemplify and clarify the difference between Assaultiveness and Tantrums. Bob's behavior (case 2) was consistent with Tantrums and was most accurately described by that term. Although David clearly did not tolerate much frustration either, the behavioral manifestation of that limitation—Assaultiveness—more accurately describes David's difficulties and, hence, was chosen preferentially for inclusion in his impairment list.

Patient: David C.

Diagnosis:

Axis I: Major Depressive Disorder, Single Episode, With Psychotic Features (296.24); Intermittent Explosive Disorder (312.24)

Axis II: None

Impairments:

1. **Delusions (Paranoid)**
2. **Assaultiveness**
3. **Dysphoric Mood**
4. **Inadequate Self-Maintenance Skills**
5. **Family Dysfunction**

* *Note to the reader: We do not use the familiar and often-used term* poor impulse control *as an impairment to describe these kinds of behaviors. Poor impulse control is a theoretical explanation of objectionable behavior based on "drive model" psychoanalytic metapsychology, and we find the term overused and often misunderstood. The question to be asked when confronted with such an "explanation" is, What happens when there is a loss of "impulse control"? The answer to that question is the basis for selecting the appropriate impairment.*

Case 6: Jerry D.

History

Jerry, a 28-year-old electrician, sought treatment for alcohol abuse and a failing marriage. He reported drinking daily since his early teens and currently drank at lunch hour, on work breaks, and nearly every evening. He attended social engagements only when alcohol was served and, more often than not, would become intoxicated. At least once a week he experienced a blackout, not remembering when or even how he got home. Jerry nervously revealed that his wife had recently moved out of the house and was threatening divorce. Since then he reported feeling very lonely, helpless about how to restore his relationship with his wife, and full of worry as to how he would ever find another "girl of my dreams." He wanted his wife to become involved in treatment with him to work on their marital problems. Jerry had tried attending Alcoholics Anonymous and even obtained a sponsor to help him develop a program of sobriety, but he was unable to stay sober. He was frightened about hospitalization but thought he needed it and did not know what else to do. His wife agreed to participate in his rehabilitation treatment program.

Clinical Presentation

Jerry presented as an attentive, polite, nicely groomed male who was motivated to save his marriage and distressed about his alcohol abuse and the effect it was having on his relationship with his wife. Although at times he felt helpless and hopeless in the face of his problem, he denied any suicidal ideation or plan. He indicated that some of his friends noticed he was withdrawing from them and that he often appeared to be sad and preoccupied. There was no evidence of a thought disorder or organic impairment.

Assessment

Although Jerry was feeling hopeless about his marital situation and it was in turn affecting his ability to work on his alcohol abuse problem, he did not meet the criteria for a DSM-IV mood disorder. Yet, he did exhibit a number of observable behaviors consistent with a Dysphoric Mood. The Substance Abuse (Alcohol) was clearly out of Jerry's control and endangering his life (the blackouts). Jerry's Dysphoric Mood was manifested by worry, feelings of sadness and futility, and his inability to concentrate (daydreaming). Even though Jerry was admitted to an inpatient alcohol rehabilitation program, the Dysphoric Mood and Marital/Relationship Dysfunction would impact the clinical course of his alcohol abuse rehabilitation and would therefore require additional, specific treatment interventions as well.

Patient: Jerry D.

Diagnosis:

Axis I: Alcohol Abuse (305.00)
Axis II: None

Impairments:

1. **Substance Abuse (Alcohol)**
2. **Dysphoric Mood**
3. **Marital/Relationship Dysfunction**

Case 7: Darryl C.

History

Darryl, an 8-year-old, was referred for psychiatric evaluation by his third-grade teacher because he was "acting odd and depressed" in the classroom. Darryl's mother accompanied him to the interview. She reported that Darryl had always been a loner, a child who preferred to be at home with her rather than with children his age. Whenever his mother had tried to encourage him to interact with anyone outside his family, Darryl would either burst into tears, saying he was afraid, or else immediately refuse and retreat to his room. His mother indicated that he appeared most happy when engaged at his computer, where he could entertain himself for hours on end and into the night with computer games, computer drawing, and science education tutorials.

Darryl had been identified as a very bright, intellectually gifted child with special interests and talent in mathematics and science. In the last year, Darryl became preoccupied with the idea that because he could learn math and science on a computer, there was no reason for him to go to school at all. He persevered in repetitive, incessant debates with his parents to convince them of this fact. His mother and father both sensed that Darryl was becoming increasingly fearful of outsiders. At times they had found him in his room crying, and on one occasion Darryl asked his mother what she thought about people who kill themselves. Darryl had one sister, 3 years younger, who appeared to be developing normally.

Clinical Presentation

Darryl presented as an unanimated, almost mannequin-like, 8-year-old who sat rigidly erect in his chair, not moving a muscle, staring directly into the interviewer's eyes. He was garrulous and very proficient in his use of language, but his speech was stilted. Darryl's "conversation" sounded more like a practice recitation in front of a mirror—how one might sound when talking to oneself.

Darryl acknowledged he often felt sad and occasionally cried but stated that he did not know the reason why. He could always make himself feel better by sitting down at his computer. He had frequent thoughts about dying but stated that he did not want to hurt his mother.

He regarded himself as intellectually superior to his peers and reported he had no interest in any of the things children his age liked to do. He felt "picked on" by his classmates but at the same time was insensitive to the provocativeness of his repeated critical attacks on them as being "intellectually inferior." Darryl was quick to add that if he were asked by anyone to do something he did not want to do (e.g., read aloud in class or play some particular game with a peer), he would become "very upset" and desperate to be in his room at his computer. He stated that he never had any use for fairy tales and found them boring.

Although Darryl was impressively knowledgeable about computer and other sciences, he was conspicuously uninformed about social norms and conventions of social interaction. The logic of his attending school rather than learning about life through a computer eluded him.

Assessment

Darryl's diagnostic formulation was tentative, and the case could be made that Darryl was demonstrating a schizophrenic disorder rather than psychotic depression and autistic behaviors. We point out here that the impairment list describes the specific manifestations of his presentation that will be addressed in treatment regardless of the patient's "final" diagnosis.

Patient: Darryl C.

Diagnosis:

Axis I: Major Depressive Disorder, Single Episode, With Psychotic Features (296.24)
Axis II: Autistic Disorder (299.00)

Impairments:

1. **Psychotic Thought/Behavior**
2. **Dysphoric Mood**
3. **Inadequate Self-Maintenance Skills**
4. **Social Withdrawal**

Case 8: Jason K.

History

Jason was an 11-year-old brought in for evaluation by his parents after he threatened to kill himself with a knife. For the last several months, Jason had been refusing to go to school and when coerced to do so would have such tantrums that it was impossible to get him out of the house. In the last several weeks, Jason would conclude his tantrums with a threat to kill himself. On the evening prior to the evaluation, his parents had discovered that Jason had a knife with him in his bed. Jason threatened that he might use it if they tried to take it away. Jason had been voicing his resistance to going to school for 2 years. He never gave any reasons for this; yet, more and more frequently, when he did go to school he would be in the school nurse's office by midmorning, in tears, complaining of a headache or a stomachache, wanting to go home. The parents felt helpless.

Jason's parents reported that he enjoyed playing baseball with his friends, as long as he was close to his home, and that he enjoyed family activities as well. On one occasion, Jason did say that he was worried some harm might befall his mother when he was not at home. Whenever Jason was asked to do something he did not want to do, he would yell, stamp his feet, strike out, throw things against the walls, kick the walls, slam doors, curse, and, most recently, threaten to kill himself.

Clinical Presentation

Jason presented as a small-for-his-age 11-year-old who clearly gave the impression of being at the evaluation under duress. His answers to questions were skimpy, at times curt. Whenever he had the opportunity to disagree, he would become vigorously vocal and animated. Several times he disagreed with his own previous statements, yet this never daunted him. He would only state that he hated school and just wanted to stay home and play. Jason denied periods of sadness or loneliness, and he denied having made statements regarding suicide or having the knife in his bed. These "disclaimers" seemed more contrary than they were dishonest or due to forgetting. There were no psychotic processes in evidence. His intellectual functioning was unimpaired.

Assessment

Even though school refusal in DSM-IV is understood as being symptomatic of a Separation Anxiety Disorder rather than a discrete disorder itself, we chose to include School Avoidance as an impairment because it is an effective descriptor of Jason's behavior (Appendix A) and is quantifiable and contains a spectrum for change that can be behaviorally measured. We chose to include both the Tantrums and the Oppositionalism because, although the Tantrums are the end result of an oppositional en-

Patient: Jason K.

Diagnosis:

Axis I: Separation Anxiety Disorder (309.21); Oppositional Defiant Disorder (313.81)

Axis II: None

Impairments:

1. **Suicidal Thought/Behavior**
2. **School Phobia**
3. **Tantrums**
4. **Oppositionalism**
5. **Family Dysfunction**

counter with an adult, Jason's arguing and defiant refusal of adult requests would require different treatment interventions (see Chapter 8) apart from and after the resolution of the Tantrums.

* *Note to the reader:* *Is Jason depressed? This is an interesting question that highlights the multiplicity of meanings of the term that are often not clarified in discussion. Are not most, if not all, actively suicidal patients depressed? That Jason is a suicide risk is clear from his behavioral presentation, and, hence, we included it in the patient impairment list. Although there is a manipulative quality to his threats of suicide, they are still desperate statements and conjure associations of helplessness and hopelessness. Yet Jason does not demonstrate any visible signs or symptoms of a Dysphoric Mood—for example, psychomotor retardation; any statements of hopelessness; or any expressions of sadness, feeling blue, or feeling lonely. Jason was not phenomenologically depressed. At the same time, we are inclined to believe that Jason's School Avoidance, Tantrums, and Oppositionalism were all attempts at mastering a "depressive core" that is the basis of a separation anxiety disorder. If, after successful treatment of the School Avoidance, Tantrums, and Oppositionalism, the "depression" is unmasked and reveals itself behaviorally, then the impairment of Dysphoric Mood may be added to Jason's impairment list (with the successfully "repaired" impairments having been deleted from it).*

Case 9: Nancy D.

Clinical Presentation

Nancy, 30 years old and single, presented at her internist's office with complaints of severe chest constriction. On examination, she was told that she had a "mild pneumonia" that could be easily treated on an outpatient basis. Nancy became irate and stormed around the room, yelling that she felt like she was going to die, terrified that her lungs might "fill up again," and that she needed to be in the hospital. She demanded to use the telephone to find another doctor who would hospitalize her. When the internist tried to reassure and calm her, she became even more agitated and left the examining room. She then began badgering the receptionist to "please get me into a hospital," screaming that no one understood how bad she felt, that she could not sit still a minute longer, and that she "had not slept in 2 days." "My legs won't stop dancing," she pleaded. Nancy was unable to process any sentences longer than four or five words because she became so agitated and distraught. She became threatening and accusing when confronted about the inappropriateness of her behavior by the receptionist, and she refused to leave the office unless she got her way. The internist then consulted a psychiatrist, and together they admitted her to a psychiatric facility. The patient's health insurance plan required preauthorization for hospitalization except in the case of medical emergency.

Assessment

This case is included to illustrate the patient impairment list as a vital, dynamic document that, when examined retrospectively, recounts the evolving evaluation and treatment process in difficult-to-diagnose cases. Nancy's severe Motor Hyperactivity and its profound interference with even the most rudimentary basic functioning argued for prompt, intensive intervention. Admitting a patient to rule out a diagnosis of a Bipolar Disorder does not communicate adequately why the patient needs treatment.

Patient: Nancy D.

Diagnosis:

Axis I: Rule Out Bipolar I Disorder, Single Manic Episode, Severe With Psychotic Features (296.04)
Axis II: None

Impairments:

1. Motor Hyperactivity

After Nancy was hospitalized, more information was obtained. Nancy had, in fact, been recently discharged from another medical facility for treatment of a pulmonary fat embolism following an outpatient surgical procedure she had had earlier that same day—hence, the fear of her lungs filling up again. While on the psychiatric unit, neurological evaluation subsequently concluded that Nancy had also probably suffered a basal ganglia infarct following the embolism, resulting in the parkinsonism that was responsible for her shuffling, agitated gait—her "dancing legs." It was also discovered that about a year prior to her psychiatric admission, she had been treated as an outpatient for a manic episode but had discontinued her medication and therapy about 4 months ago. Once the explanation for her Motor Hyperactivity was found, Nancy's impairment list was revised.

Impairments (updated):

1. **Motor Hyperactivity (Revised: see 2, 3, 4)**
2. **Manic Thought/Behavior**
3. **Concomitant Medical Condition (parkinsonism, secondary to basal ganglia infarct, posttraumatic)**
4. **Medication Treatment Noncompliance**

Case 10: Richard J.

Clinical Presentation

Richard, a 29-year-old married construction worker, sought treatment to repair a failing marriage. He indicated that his wife had threatened to leave him, and, when faced with this possibility, he found himself becoming increasingly irritable. Richard also began to dread what life would be like without her and felt anxious that life might "never be the same." He was angry that his wife was spending more and more time away from home and complained accusingly that she was now consuming alcohol almost daily. He acknowledged that he also drank daily, "but not as much as she did."

His wife, Carolyn, reported a long history of struggling with her husband to improve their communication. She stated that from the beginning of their 6-year marriage he would frequently work late into the evening, often failing to keep his promise to call her when he knew this was going to occur. She stated that they quickly lost the common friends and interests they shared prior to getting married. As a result, she began spending more and more time with single friends from work and, in the last few months, had on occasion drunk until she either passed out or blacked out. Two weeks ago, she decided to take the advice of friends and attended several Alcoholics Anonymous meetings. At the time of the interview, she had 1 week of sobriety. She felt that to be successful with her sobriety plan it was important for her husband never to drink in her presence. She also wondered whether the marriage was salvageable because she was not sure if she cared anymore. The years of trying to make her husband pay attention to her and the years of trying to have a social life without her husband had left her distant from him, and she did not want to be hurt and unhappy anymore.

Assessment

Richard actually sought treatment because of despondent concerns about his failing marriage that were causing him a great deal of anxiety. His diagnoses do not completely and accurately communicate the nature of his difficulties—which an outside reviewer would need to know before authorizing marital therapy for him. Whether he had a primary alcohol abuse problem at the time of the initial evaluation was unclear; however, his drinking was clearly compounding the marital difficulties and, as a result, increasing his agitation and worry about the future, hence its inclusion as an impairment.

Patient: Richard J.

Diagnosis:

Axis I: Atypical Depression (311)
Axis II: Alcohol Abuse (305.00)

Impairments:

1. **Anxiety**
2. **Substance Abuse (Alcohol)**
3. **Marital/Relationship Dysfunction**

* *Note to the reader: Had Richard's wife been the problematic drinker instead, the impairment Marital/Relationship Dysfunction With Substance Abuse would have replaced Marital/Relationship Dysfunction and Substance Abuse (Alcohol).*

Case 11: Beatrice D.

History

Beatrice, 73 years old, was referred for evaluation by the owners of the board and care facility where she resided because "she's talking to imaginary people, physically attacking her roommate without apparent provocation, and refusing to eat or take her high blood pressure pills." She had resided there for 7 years, had never been a management problem, and took no other medications. Also, Beatrice's personal hygiene had become increasingly poor over the last several months. No other information was available at the time of evaluation.

Clinical Presentation

Beatrice presented as an elderly, unkempt, disheveled, adequately nourished, well-hydrated female who was visibly suspiciously and furtively looking about the room. Her speech was fluent, and she shouted repeatedly that she was being "taken away from my home." She blamed her caregivers for all her current difficulties. She was excitable and at times refused to talk. Beatrice refused to answer any questions regarding her mood, folding her arms across her chest and staring away from the interviewer. She did state, however, that several "little people" had been coming into her room now and then and occasionally moved and rearranged her furniture and belongings. She did not mind that, however, and said she enjoyed talking to her "little friends." She acknowledged becoming irate whenever anyone else came into her room—"They were stepping on my little friends!"—and she felt the need to protect her little friends by pummeling her intruders. She also reported hearing voices but did not know from where they came. They were male voices and usually just called her name. Beatrice did not know the date, the day of the week, or the month. She became angry when asked her address or the name of the facility where she was residing. Beatrice knew her birthday. When asked to remember the names of two unrelated objects, after a few minutes of distraction, she could not recall them. She could recall three numbers forward and two numbers backward. Blood pressure was 180/100, pulse was 80 and irregular, and she was afebrile.

Assessment

Beatrice was obviously psychotic, a danger to others, and unable to care for herself. The reasons for this in the absence of any psychiatric history were unclear. Her elevated blood pressure was probably the result of her lack of compliance with her medical regimen. Beatrice was admitted to the hospital for medical, neurological, and psychiatric evaluation.

Patient: Beatrice D.

Diagnosis:

Axis I: Delirium Not Otherwise Specified (780.09)
Axis II: Deferred

Impairments:

1. **Hallucinations**
2. **Assaultiveness**
3. **Inadequate Healthcare Skills**
4. **Medical Treatment Noncompliance**

* *Note to the reader:* *This case is included to illustrate a not unfamiliar clinical presentation that is often subject to more rigorous review. Subsequent neurological evaluation concluded that Beatrice was suffering from Alzheimer's disease (ICD-9-CM 331.0 [World Health Organization 1980]), which would be coded on Axis III. A diagnosis of Delirium or Dementia suggests to reviewers the presence of an "organic brain syndrome," which, in turn, suggests chronicity. A chronic condition does not by itself justify acute care. We used the patient impairment list to structure the communication of the acuity of Beatrice's difficulties. In this particular case, we prefer to use the impairments of Hallucinations and Assaultiveness rather than Psychotic Thought/Behavior because the former are the more specific, accurate descriptors of her difficulties that necessitated treatment.*

Case 12: Peter K.

History

Peter, a 45-year-old bus driver, had recently moved from another state to his present residence. After the move, he sought out a new psychiatrist, who gave him chlorpromazine, which he had been taking since his last psychiatric hospitalization 2 years earlier. Peter had had seven hospitalizations for acute schizophrenic episodes since the age of 19. In the acute phases of his illness, he would become extremely paranoid, delusionally jealous, severely agitated, and on three occasions physically threatening. Peter described his behavior during these episodes as "very bizarre." For the last 2 years, he has maintained himself on chlorpromazine, 200 mg a day, without relapse. He has been able to work full-time as a bus driver for the city's transportation department and takes good care of his personal and financial responsibilities. He has lived alone since moving out of his parents' home when he was 24. Peter was able to identify the specific social situations that made him feel paranoid and fearful of "having crazy thoughts and losing control" again, so he avoided them as much as possible. He acknowledged he occasionally had difficulty determining how much of his feeling persecuted was real and wished to know how much additional chlorpromazine he might need to take and for how long.

Assessment

Although Peter's condition is in remission at this time, he still considers psychotherapy treatment to be necessary to help him continue to sort out what is real and not real, both in his thoughts and in his perceptions. He also notes that the medication is particularly helpful when he begins to feel paranoid, and he titrates this symptom with an additional 50–150 mg of chlorpromazine a day. The impairments clearly communicate to any reviewer the two areas of difficulty that require both ongoing psychotherapy and medication maintenance management.

Patient: Peter K.

Diagnosis:

Axis I: Schizophrenia, Paranoid Type, Unspecified Pattern (295.30)
Axis II: None

Impairments:

1. **Delusions (Paranoid)**
2. **Psychotic Thought/Behavior**

* *Note to the reader: Because there are two clinical issues to be addressed in the treatment—namely, the chronic feelings of being persecuted (with which he continually struggles) and the periodic episodes of bizarre thoughts and behavior—both the Delusions and the Psychotic Thought/Behavior are identified in the patient impairment list.*

Conclusion

After the justification for treatment is established, the practitioner needs to provide convincing information to support the type and intensity of treatment being recommended for the patient. The usefulness of the impairment list for structuring this discussion with reviewers and documenting the question, How sick is the patient? is the subject of Chapter 6.

Chapter 6

Impairment Severity and the Appropriateness of Treatment

"Can the patient be treated at a lower level of care?"

The assignment of severity-of-illness ratings to acute medical-surgical care diagnoses is now a legislative mandate in many states. Severity ratings can also be determined for each impairment, based on specific patient statements and behaviors. We describe five degrees of severity that are used to rate selected "critical" impairments; all impairments may be rated with the three lower levels of severity.

The patient vignettes presented in Chapter 5 illustrate the utility of the impairment language for communicating and documenting convincing reasons why a patient seeks (or requires) mental health treatment. In addition to establishing that treatment is *necessary*, the practitioner is also responsible for justifying that the recommended treatment is *appropriate*. In our experience with inpatient facilities and managed care review organizations, a majority of reimbursement denials are the result of inadequate (or absent) articulation of a convincing rationale or justification as to *why* the patient requires the (additional) care. Appropriateness is a cardinal concern for purchasers of healthcare. In the absence of a universal definition for appropriate care, we employ two: 1) appropriateness is "the degree to which the care provided is relevant to the patient's clinical needs, given the current state of knowledge" (Joint Commission on Accreditation of Healthcare Organizations 1994, p. 42), and 2) care is appropriate when the benefits of treatment outweigh the risks and are worth the cost. The impairment language is the basis for a treatment documentation method that convincingly conveys appropriateness of care to those who need to know.

Convincing a managed care reviewer that an intensive treatment approach (e.g., weekly psychotherapy and monthly medication management) is more appropriate than, say, monthly medication monitoring alone is an often frustrating obligation for the practitioner. We have been able to intercede on behalf of practitioners and reverse successfully a number of denials for care once *we* understood from the practitioner why the treatment was appropriate. To do this, we ask two questions: 1) How serious is the patient's problem? and 2) What will the patient say or do to evidence that the treatment is working?

Both this chapter on impairment severity and Chapter 7, in which we address patient objectives, describe a procedure the practitioner can use to convey clinical necessity and appropriateness of the proposed treatment effectively, as well as justify being paid for it.

Severity of Illness

Severity of illness describes the degree of risk of immediate death or permanent loss of function due to a disease (or impairment). The term *case complexity* is also now being employed to address severity of illness, although these two concepts are not quite the same. Patients who are "complex" (i.e., have multiple impairments or a complicated impairment profile) may or may not be severely ill with respect to immediate risk of death or permanent loss of function. Therefore, we shall adhere to the severity-of-illness concept (for our purposes, the severity of the impairment) as it relates to the clinical appropriateness of care.

The current diagnosis-related group (DRG) Medicare Prospective Payment System (PPS) does not adequately take severity of illness into account. As a result, hospitals that treat a greater proportion of more severely ill patients may sometimes "appear" to have higher costs, lower productivity, and poorer quality of care, when actually the explanation lies in the fact that their patient population may be genuinely sicker. Severely ill patients are often critically ill and require more costly care in intensive care units. A real concern is that some hospitals might have to refuse to treat these sicker patients if DRG payments do not cover treatment costs. One solution to this dilemma has been to adjust the DRGs with an appropriate severity-of-illness measure so that critically ill patients are appropriately classified, cared for, and paid for. The Yale School of Management, under a Health Care Financing Administration contract, has developed a system called the DRG refinement algorithm to do this. The DRG refinement condenses the currently used 475 DRGs into approximately 385 "refined groups," each of which has either three or four severity levels. However, as this edition goes to press, the Health Care Financing Administration still has not received congressional approval to adopt the DRG refinement for use with the Medicare PPS.

There is another line in the historical development of the current concepts of severity of illness with which mental healthcare practitioners should be familiar. After the implementation of the Medicare PPS, it became possible for hospitals to combine clinical patient information and financial information (charge data) for studying the appropriateness of hospital use (utilization), for improving charge comparisons across hospitals and departments within hospitals, and for strategically planning budgets. Several major accounting firms developed automated "case mix" management systems to help hospitals do this. Medicare patients' DRGs were matched with charge data to compare practitioner utilization of resources and ordering practices. The objection was immediately raised, of course, that some practitioners' patients were receiving more resources because they were "sicker"—that is, more severely ill. Unless these more severely ill patients were identified and the degree of their severity factored into the monitoring data, accurate determinations of appropriate practitioner utilization would continue to require in-depth, time-consuming, and costly manual review of each case and each practitioner.

To fill the need for severity-adjusted utilization monitoring and to facilitate compliance with the requirement of the Joint Commission that hospitals and medical staffs perform continuous "performance improvement," as well as peer review, activities, more than a half-dozen companies have developed computerized severity-of-illness systems that can be used to evaluate clinical data and then assign each case an arbitrary severity score or rating. In several of the more widely used systems, the scores range from 0 (i.e., no significant clinical findings or complications) to 4 (i.e., critical findings indicating the presence of organ failure or death). In some systems, an additional severity level of 5 is used to signify death. At this time, there is no gold standard against which each of these severity systems can be functionally measured and evaluated. The severities of the illnesses are defined somewhat differently in each of these systems. Each system uses its own scales, which are not comparable across systems. Each system also has different fixed and variable costs. Notwithstanding the absence of the last word in severity-of-illness determination, at least 19 state legislatures have already proceeded to mandate that their hospitals' published charge data be adjusted for severity of illness (using a particular severity-of-illness system that each state chose on its own) to obtain comparative cost and quality information for all the hospitals and practitioners located in their state.

Severity of Impairments

While mental healthcare services continue to operate under a DRG exemption, three of the medical severity-of-illness systems we reviewed do contain severity criteria for the nervous and mental diseases found in the *International Classification of Diseases, 9th Revision, Clinical Modification* (ICD-9-CM) (World Health Organization 1980). The same concerns we detailed in Chapter 4 regarding the utility of the DSM-IV (American Psychiatric Association 1994) diagnoses for communicating the nature of the patient's difficulties apply when trying to use ICD-9-CM diagnoses (with which the DSM-IV is designed to be compatible) to compare their severities. Does a "very severe" Delusional Disorder, Persecutory Type (297.1—DSM-IV) require the same or similar treatment services as a "very severe" Posttraumatic Stress Disorder With Delayed Onset (309.81—DSM-IV)? The answer, of course, is a definitive "Well, maybe . . . and maybe not, too." Nonetheless, we believe that the severity-of-illness concept is relevant for determining appropriateness of mental healthcare services.

Although not a steadfast rule, generally the more severe an acute illness is, the more costly it will be to return the patient to wellness. To investigate whether this is true for the impairments, we have applied the severity-of-illness concept to the impairment language.[1] All managed care review organizations have either developed their own or adapted others' criteria linking severity and service. These appropriateness criteria—which become a review organization's "rules of the trade"—are often referred to as severity of illness/intensity of service—or "SI/IS" (InterQual terminology)—reviewer guidelines (InterQual 1993). The basic premise is that disease severity based on predetermined parameters of extent of dysfunction predetermines what treatment is necessary and appropriate. In the absence of definitive clinical outcomes research that links impairments to process, however, such criteria are only the opinions of their authors and consultants and cannot, and should not, serve as practice guidelines for practitioners.

There is much confusion about *intensity of service* and *level of care.* These terms are not synonyms for each other. For the purposes of discussion in this book, level of care refers only to treatment setting (i.e., the facility, the room, the philosophy of the treater or the treatment program). Intensity of service takes into account at least five components: personnel cost/hour, personnel/patient ratio, number of personnel hours, setting, and ancillary costs. Two patients in the same treatment setting (e.g., day treatment substance abuse program) may have very different service needs (e.g., one patient may require additional intensive marital therapy and daily physical therapy whereas another may not).

The practitioner is once again bewildered because there appear to be as many different criteria sets and treatment guidelines predetermining

---

[1] Until an impairment-based treatment database is aggregated for research analysis, this question will, of course, remain unanswered.

what is appropriate treatment as there are utilization and managed care review organizations who rely on them. The challenge for the practitioner is not to decode an organization's SI/IS (or some other set of) criteria; the task is to convey convincingly the nature, seriousness, and extent of a patient's difficulties as part of the clinical rationale for the recommended treatment.

Impairment Severity Ratings

We identify five degrees of severity to be consistent with the most widely used medical severity-of-illness systems currently employed throughout the country. These impairment severity ratings are identified by a number and its descriptor:

Severity 4: Imminently Dangerous
Severity 3: Severely Incapacitating
Severity 2: Destabilizing
Severity 1: Distressing
Severity 0: Absent or Nonpathological

A severity 4 describes an impairment that is *imminently dangerous* because either it is predictably destructive to oneself or others or totally interferes with the ability to care for oneself in any way. Behavioral examples include

- Active suicide threats or behavior
- Active violent or destructive behavior
- Active life-endangering runaway behavior or risk
- Total inability (> 90%) to perform self-care skills

A severity 3 defines an impairment that is *severely incapacitating* either because it is a potential and likely danger to oneself or others, or because it severely compromises the ability to care for oneself. Behavioral examples include

- Recent suicide behavior, threat, or current active ideation with a plan
- Recent violent or destructive behavior or current active ideation with a plan
- Recent endangering runaway behavior or current active ideation with a plan

- Severely compromised (61%–90%) ability to care for daily personal, family, financial, or employment-/school-related matters

A severity 2 defines an impairment that is *destabilizing* and, as a result, either markedly compromises (30%–60%) independent, vocational, or community functioning or inhibits the effectiveness of the treatment or the family-social support systems for "repairing" the patient's impairment.

A severity 1 defines an impairment that is *distressing* and, as a result, either compromises (< 30%) independent, vocational, community, or school- or work-related functioning or, although absent at the present time, has a predictable likelihood of occurrence or recurrence without treatment.

A severity 0 defines an impairment that is either *absent* (the impairment that has been completely "repaired") or, if present, is *nonpathological.* The 0 rating is actually an important marker for tracking the patient's progress in treatment. (This is addressed in detail in Chapter 9.)

The presence of any one or more of these global generic behaviors justifies the corresponding severity rating for that particular impairment. In most cases, these definers require elaboration and "translation" into *specific* patient statements and behaviors to justify a particular severity rating for an impairment. We emphasize that these severity ratings do not necessarily predict a particular treatment setting or intensity of service. An impairment with a severity 4 may or may not require an intensive inpatient care setting. Outpatient crisis management models may be equally effective and appropriate. Justifying a treatment setting or intensity of service requires additional information regarding the expectations of the treatment—the patient objectives—which is the subject of Chapter 7.

Critical Impairments

All of the impairments may potentially be "distressing" or "destabilizing" for a patient (severity 1 or 2). A subgroup of impairments have the potential to justify more intensive service interventions (e.g., hospitalization). Impairments in this subgroup may become either "severely incapacitating" or "imminently dangerous" (severity 3 or 4), and we refer to those impairments as "critical impairments." It should be noted that some impairments may seem to become more severe when, in fact, the explanation is the presence or emergence of another (usually critical) impairment.

Some examples should clarify this point.

If a patient whose personal hygiene skills are deteriorating (Inadequate Healthcare Skills) subsequently develops Delusions that place someone in critical danger (an elderly diabetic patient, for example, develops delusional ideation of immortality and hence, permanently cured of diabetes, no longer requires insulin), the Delusions place the patient in imminent danger (severity 4). The danger is in the Delusions, not in the Inadequate Healthcare Skills. Should the patient's poor self-care result in a diabetic coma requiring that the patient be hospitalized, the impairment of Concomitant Medical Condition is also identified as the critical impairment (and most likely rated at severity 4). If the impairment of Tantrums manifests with verbalized threats to physically harm others, Assaultiveness is identified as the potentially dangerous impairment. In the course of treatment, one can imagine that the Assaultiveness may be resolved, but treatment efforts to eliminate the Tantrums continue for sometime thereafter.

In our experience, patients who have one or more critical impairments will also have one or more noncritical impairments. Including these in the impairment list is still important for two reasons: 1) their presence often impacts treatment of the critical impairments and may help explain why progress is less rapid than might otherwise be anticipated, and 2) noncritical impairments also require treatment—even in a more costly treatment setting warranted by the presence of the critical impairments.

The practitioner is cautioned to avoid "stuffing" the patient's clinical record with impairments and severities in an effort to add weight for establishing clinical need for treatment. It is not the number of impairments but rather the impairment with the highest severity rating that will influence reviewers. There is no severity in number of impairments. A patient may have only one impairment but, with sufficient behavioral documentation of the severity level of that impairment, may be justifiably treated in a very secure intensive setting.

The impairments that have the potential to be critical are listed in Table 6–1.

Describing Impairment Severity

Practitioners intuitively make severity assessments all the time. Deciding whether an impairment is imminently dangerous, severely incapacitating, destabilizing, or distressing is a conclusion (often with an implied prediction) the practitioner makes based on

- Patient statements
- Patient behaviors
- Practitioner training
- Practitioner clinical skill
- Practitioner experience

Not dissimilar to the expert-witness opinion utilized in courts of law, a severity rating determination is the synthesis of the practitioner's education, practical knowledge, expertise, and informed observation of the patient.

Another aphorism familiar to Medicare reviewers reminds healthcare professionals, "In God we trust—all others must document!" Severity determinations must be corroborated—justified—with convincing evidence. In our experience, the most convincing evidence comes from the patient—specifically, what the patient *says* or what the patient *does*. This "say/do" model also defines the formation of patient objectives (described in Chapter 7), which, when coupled with severity ratings, convey the clinical rationale for the treatment.

To assist practitioners with this task, we have provided a reference list of impairment severity qualifiers—or "prompts"—for the four severity ratings of the critical impairments (Appendix B). Each prompt implies or suggests a patient statement or behavior that is consistent with and supports the corresponding severity rating. It is important to remember that severity ratings describe impairments the patient has—and not the pa-

Table 6–1. Critical impairments

Anxiety	Manic Thought/Behavior
Assaultiveness	Medical Risk Factor
Compulsions	Mood Lability
Concomitant Medical Condition	Obsessions
Delusions (Nonparanoid)	Phobia
Delusions (Paranoid)	Physical Abuse Perpetrator
Dissociative States	Psychomotor Retardation
Dysphoric Mood	Psychotic Thought/Behavior
Eating Disorder	Running Away
Fire Setting	Self-Mutilation
Hallucinations	Sexual Trauma Perpetrator
Homicidal Thought/Behavior	Substance Abuse
Inadequate Healthcare Skills	Suicidal Thought/Behavior

tient. If a patient has three identified impairments, each impairment has its own severity rating.

When conveying to a reviewer (or documenting in the patient record) the severity of an impairment, all that is necessary to include are the specific ratings (e.g., Dysphoric Mood, severity 2, destabilizing) and one or two corroborating statements—either a patient quote or a patient behavior. The severity qualifiers listed for the critical impairments in Appendix B are intended to prompt the practitioner to provide this kind of convincing evidence. For example, a qualifier for Dysphoric Mood, severity 2, such as "markedly compromises (30%–60%) work performance [and] ability to care for oneself," might prompt the practitioner to document: "The patient said, 'I've been at least 2 hours late for work every day this week,' and the patient is very unkempt and looks poorly groomed."

It is important to reiterate that the statements and behaviors to support impairment severity are the patient's and not the treater's. Information such as "the patient requires one-to-one supervision" or "patient needs an adequate blood level of the antidepressant" does not corroborate severity or justify a particular treatment setting. These statements are, in fact, interventions to be implemented *because* of the severity of the patient's impairments. As repeated throughout this book, managed care reviewers need to know not only what the proposed care plan for the patient will be, but also why the treatment is necessary.

✻ *Two notes of caution: First, the impairment severity qualifiers provided in Appendix B are not criteria to be met for a specific severity, nor do they constitute the only appropriate features of a patient's presentation for that rating. These qualifiers are only prompts or suggestions to which the practitioner can refer when seeking to justify a particular severity for an impairment. A patient may make statements or demonstrate behaviors that do not relate to any of these prompts. If, in the practitioner's opinion, this say/do evidence justifies a certain severity rating, then of course it should be incorporated. Second, an often-asked question is, "When a patient has, for example, two impairments with severity 3—and one with severity 4—does that make the patient a 4?" Remember that a severity rating describes the impairment and not the patient, and the decision regarding the most appropriate treatment setting usually hinges on the most severe impairment. If one is compelled to give an "overall" severity descriptor, we recommend that it be the severity of the impairment with the highest rating.*

The patient's impairments that are prioritized as the focus of treatment and their respective severity ratings constitute a patient impairment profile (PIP).

Case Examples

Two patient vignettes are presented to illustrate the application of severity ratings to the impairments. In the interest of brevity, the discussion of these two cases focuses only on determining the severity ratings for the critical impairments. The severity rating qualifiers for both patients' critical impairments are included. We apply the patient's clinical presentation (i.e., what the patient said or did) to the severity prompts and determine the appropriate severity ratings for each impairment.

We continue to use the case examples of Melanie W. and Bob D., introduced in Chapter 5, because they are particularly instructive and illustrative. These cases are the clinical examples also used in subsequent chapters to demonstrate the use of the PIP for selecting patient objectives and specifying the target objectives (Chapter 7), generating a treatment plan (Chapter 8), and tracking the patient's progress in treatment (Chapter 9).

Case 1: Melanie W.

Case 1: Melanie W.

Impairments:

1. **Suicidal Thought/Behavior**
2. **Dysphoric Mood**
3. **Concomitant Medical Condition (juvenile-type diabetes mellitus)**
4. **Inadequate Healthcare Skills**
5. **Family Dysfunction**
6. **Truancy**

Severity Qualifiers for Suicidal Thought/Behavior:

Severity 4: Imminently Dangerous

- Places self in immediate, life-threatening danger.
- Patient has unremitting intent to commit suicide.
- Patient has made a recent life-threatening suicide attempt.
- Patient actively plans lethal suicide attempts daily.
- Totally interferes (> 90%) with the ability to care for oneself.

Severity 3: Severely Incapacitating

- Places self or others in likely danger.
- Patient has active suicide plans that are prevented up to 8 hours using a signed agreement to that effect.
- Recent history of dangerous suicide attempt.
- Active suicide plans or suicide gestures daily.
- Severely interferes (61%–90%) with the ability to care for oneself.

Severity 2: Destabilizing

- Suicide ideation or plan present at least weekly.
- Patient has active suicide plans that are prevented up to 24 hours using a signed agreement to that effect.
- Past history (> 3 months ago) of suicide attempt or recent history of active suicide plans.
- Patient can interrupt Suicidal Thought/Behavior only with intensive therapeutic support.

Severity 1: Distressing

- Suicide ideation present.
- Patient has a history of one or more suicide gestures or nonlethal attempts.
- Patient can interrupt Suicidal Thought/Behavior only with frequent therapeutic support.

Severity Qualifiers for Dysphoric Mood:

Severity 4: Imminently Dangerous

- Places self or others in immediate, life-threatening danger.
- Present more than 75% of the day.
- Totally interferes (> 90%) with the ability to care for oneself.
- Totally interferes (> 90%) with:
    - carrying out daily personal, family, financial, or legal responsibilities,

or

following a prescribed treatment regimen.

Severity 3: Severely Incapacitating

- Places self or others in likely danger.
- Severely interferes (61%–90%) with the ability to care for oneself.
- Severely interferes (61%–90%) with:

  carrying out daily personal, family, financial, or legal responsibilities,

  or

  performing complex/new tasks at work/school,

  or

  following a prescribed treatment regimen.

Severity 2: Destabilizing

- Present more than 25% of the day.
- Markedly interferes (30%–60%) with the ability to care for oneself.
- Markedly interferes (30%–60%) with:

  carrying out daily personal, family, financial, or legal responsibilities,

  or

  performing complex/new tasks at work/school,

  or

  following a prescribed treatment regimen.
- Patient requires intensive therapeutic support to interrupt the Dysphoric Mood.

Severity 1: Distressing

- Present daily to weekly.
- Compromises (< 30%) optimal ability to care for oneself.
- Compromises (< 30%) optimal ability to:

  carry out daily personal, family, financial, or legal responsibilities,

  or

  perform complex/new tasks at work/school,

  or

  follow a prescribed treatment regimen.
- Patient requires frequent therapeutic support to interrupt Dysphoric Mood.

Severity Qualifiers for Concomitant Medical Condition:

Severity 4: Imminently Dangerous

- Life threatening for the patient.
- Patient totally unable or unwilling to manage the Concomitant Medical Condition.
- Totally interferes (> 90%) with the ability to care for oneself.

Severity 3: Severely Incapacitating

- Dangerous but not imminently life threatening for the patient.
- Patient denies extent of the Concomitant Medical Condition.
- Patient denies potential dangerous consequences of inadequate management of the Concomitant Medical Condition.

Severity 2: Destabilizing

- Concomitant Medical Condition is unstable.
- Patient management of the Concomitant Medical Condition is medically unacceptable.

Severity 1: Distressing

- Concomitant Medical Condition requires regular medical supervision.
- Patient verbalizes distress about the presence of the Concomitant Medical Condition.

The reader will recall from Chapter 5 that 17-year-old Melanie, believing that she had no future for herself, had verbalized the desire to die. She had stated that she had found an easy way of killing herself: by eating all the sugars she wanted to and not taking her insulin or by injecting herself with too much insulin. She talked about going to the corner store, buying chocolate bars, and "eating chocolate and getting drunk to have a good time before I die." Melanie fantasized about being in a diabetic coma, dying, with the ambulance arriving minutes too late. She knew the times of the day and locations to go where she would not be found until it was too late. Melanie was habitually truant and spent most of her days at home taking care of her younger siblings, who were largely neglected by both parents.

The Suicidal Thought/Behavior in Melanie's PIP was rated at severity 4. Melanie's intentional manipulation of her insulin repeatedly placed her in serious medical danger. Excessive or inadequate insulin administration could be lethal for her, and Melanie's unwillingness to follow a prescribed insulin regimen placed her at high risk. About a year ago, Melanie had also cut both of her wrists with a razor blade deep enough to necessitate suturing. (After Melanie's referral for a psychiatric evaluation, she was hospitalized in an acute psychiatric unit.)

The Dysphoric Mood in Melanie's PIP was rated at severity 4. Melanie's personal hygiene was very poor (e.g., dirty hair, unwashed face, and wrinkled and soiled clothes). She verbalized that she did not care how she looked or what others thought of her. Most of Melanie's statements were self-critical, with expressions of hopelessness and thoughts of suicide. She felt totally helpless in trying to solve her very real family problems, and she was overwhelmed with the self-assigned responsibility of caring for her siblings that she (accurately) felt was necessary, given her parents' deficiencies, ineffectiveness, and unavailability.

Melanie had no desire to attend school and when forced to go was unable to concentrate or complete any assignments. She usually would leave by third period. Melanie often daydreamed, not listening to conversations with teachers or friends, and felt distracted even in her favorite pastime, watching television. She reported a loss of desire to be around people. Being with friends or shopping with her mother no longer was fun. She preferred to hide in her room. The only pleasure she experienced was when intoxicated by alcohol. Melanie also verbalized that she did not have the energy or the desire to try any of the suggestions made by family, friends, medical doctors, or therapists. Her answer, "Why bother!" had ceased to be a question.

Initially, the Concomitant Medical Condition in Melanie's PIP was rated at severity 4. Without proper medical management, Melanie was at critical risk for a number of the life-threatening complications of untreated diabetes mellitus. She required acute medical care (hospitalization) to be stabilized. Melanie had been refusing to monitor her blood glucose levels prior to hospitalization, and, although she was well educated as to how to do so, her overall management of her diabetes was very poor.

Melanie's initial PIP (both impairments and severity ratings) follows:

Case 1: Melanie W.

Patient Impairment Profile

Impairment	Severity
1. **Suicidal Thought/Behavior**	4
2. **Dysphoric Mood**	4
3. **Concomitant Medical Condition (juvenile-type diabetes mellitus)**	4
4. **Inadequate Healthcare Skills**	2
5. **Family Dysfunction**	2
6. **Truancy**	2

Case 2: Bob D.

Case 2: Bob D.

Impairments:

1. **Delusions (Nonparanoid)**
2. **Substance Abuse (Alcohol)**
3. **Tantrums**

Severity Qualifiers for Delusions (Nonparanoid):

Severity 4: Imminently Dangerous

- Places self or others in immediate, life-threatening danger.
- Unremitting delusional thinking.
- Patient convinced Delusions are true and acts accordingly.
- Totally interferes (> 90%) with the ability to care for oneself.
- Totally interferes (> 90%) with:

  carrying out daily personal, family, financial, or legal responsibilities,

  or

  following a prescribed treatment regimen.
- Confrontation about the Delusions increases anxiety, further impairing ability to function.

Severity 3: Severely Incapacitating

- Places self or others in likely danger.
- Preoccupation with Delusions at least half the time.
- Patient believes Delusions are true but does not act on them.
- Severely interferes (61%–90%) with the ability to care for oneself.
- Severely interferes (61%–90%) with:
  carrying out daily personal, family, financial, or legal responsibilities,
  or
  performing complex/new tasks at work/school,
  or
  following a prescribed treatment regimen.

Severity 2: Destabilizing

- Patient unsure if Delusions are true.
- Present daily to weekly.
- Markedly interferes (30%–60%) with the ability to care for oneself.
- Markedly interferes (30%–60%) with:
  carrying out daily personal, family, financial, or legal responsibilities,
  or
  performing complex/new tasks at work/school,
  or
  following a prescribed treatment regimen.
- Markedly disruptive (> 30%) to the daily functioning of others.

Severity 1: Distressing

- Patient able to consider alternative explanations for delusional thinking.
- Compromises (< 30%) optimal ability to care for oneself.
- Compromises (< 30%) optimal ability to:
  carry out daily personal, family, financial, or legal responsibilities,
  or
  perform complex/new tasks at work/school,
  or
  follow a prescribed treatment regimen.
- Compromises (> 30%) the optimal daily functioning of others.

Severity Qualifiers for Substance Abuse:

Severity 4: Imminently Dangerous

- Places self or others in immediate, life-threatening danger.
- Patient has been abusing substances for at least 4 weeks—cessation of which places the patient at high risk for a life-threatening physical withdrawal syndrome.
- Totally interferes (> 90%) with the ability to care for oneself.
- Totally interferes (> 90%) with:

  carrying out daily personal, family, financial, or legal responsibilities,

  or

  following a prescribed treatment regimen.
- Patient has a history of one or more episodes of life-threatening alcohol/drug withdrawal.
- Patient has a Concomitant Medical Condition that is imminently dangerous (severity 4).
- Patient has another psychiatric impairment that is imminently dangerous (severity 4).

Severity 3: Severely Incapacitating

- Places self or others in likely danger.
- Patient has been abusing substances for the last 4 weeks—cessation of which places the patient at risk for withdrawal.
- Patient is unable to maintain abstinence for 24 hours without around-the-clock supervision.
- Severely interferes (61%–90%) with the ability to care for oneself.
- Severely interferes (61%–90%) with:

  carrying out daily personal, family, financial, or legal responsibilities,

  or

  performing complex/new tasks at work/school,

  or

  following a prescribed treatment regimen.
- Patient has a history of two or more failures of detoxification at less intensive levels of care.
- Patient has a Concomitant Medical Condition that is incapacitating (severity 3).

- Patient has another psychiatric impairment that is incapacitating (severity 3).
- Patient's previous efforts to maintain abstinence have been actively sabotaged by either:
  family or significant other,
  or
  occupation or social setting.

Severity 2: Destabilizing

- Patient is unable to maintain abstinence while participating in a treatment program for more than 3 months without relapsing.
- Patient is unable to maintain abstinence for more than 3 months following completion of an outpatient program.
- Markedly interferes (30%–60%) with:
  carrying out daily personal, family, financial, or legal responsibilities,
  or
  performing complex/new tasks at work/school,
  or
  following a prescribed treatment regimen.
- Patient has a Concomitant Medical Condition that is destabilizing (severity 2).
- Patient has another psychiatric impairment that is destabilizing (severity 2).
- Patient's current treatment is likely to be interfered with or potentially sabotaged by either:
  family or significant other,
  or
  occupation or social setting.

Severity 1: Distressing

- Patient requires regular therapeutic support to maintain abstinence.
- Compromises (< 30%) optimal ability to:
  carry out daily personal, family, financial, or legal responsibilities,
  or
  perform complex/new tasks at work/school,

or

follow a prescribed treatment regimen.

- Patient has a Concomitant Medical Condition that is distressing (severity 1).
- Patient has another psychiatric impairment that is distressing (severity 1).
- Compromises the optimal daily functioning of others.

Bob's clinical presentation is detailed in Chapter 5 and is only summarized here. Bob, a 23-year-old white married male, was brought to an emergency room by his parents for an acute episode of delusional behavior and acute alcohol intoxication. Bob presented with bizarre religious beliefs that he felt gave him the right and power to break into buildings, claim them as God's, and then demolish them to appropriate the land for children's parks. Married for just over a year, Bob had never settled into a job in which he felt comfortable. He had been observed on many occasions to be easily angered when he did not get his way or anyone disagreed with him. He would "kick and scream like a small child." His friends and family had no more patience for his immaturity.

The Delusions in Bob's PIP were rated at severity 4. The Delusions confirmed his right to break into buildings, placing him (and perhaps others) in imminent danger. In this regard, he demonstrated a total absence of judgment and was unable to care for himself. He was at times too preoccupied with his own delusional beliefs to listen accurately or to concentrate, let alone follow any treatment recommendations or perform any complex or varied tasks. (Bob was, in fact, admitted to the intensive care unit of a psychiatric hospital.)

The Substance Abuse (Alcohol) in Bob's PIP was rated at severity 4 at the time of admission. The question was raised as to whether the delusional disorder was the result of alcohol or some other drug intoxication. Regardless of the cause, however, the Delusions placed Bob in imminent danger because of their content. With a reported daily intake of six to eight beers, the possibility of his drinking much more than that and the possibility of his having a life-threatening physical withdrawal were active treatment concerns. Certainly at the time of admission, Bob was totally unable to take care of himself. Finally, his frequent Tantrums had just about depleted the patience of his friends and family. As a result, his support system was deteriorating and with it any stability he may have had in the past. The Tantrums were now destabilizing for Bob—hence the rating at severity 2.

Bob's initial PIP (impairments and severity ratings) follows:

Case 2: Bob D.

Patient Impairment Profile

Impairment	Severity
1. Delusions	4
2. Substance Abuse (Alcohol)	4
3. Tantrums	2

On the second day of hospitalization, it was established that Bob had actually been experiencing a phencyclidine (PCP)-induced delusional disorder. By that time, the delusional disorder had run its course, and there was no evidence of alcohol withdrawal thus far. No further evidence could be found to establish an alcohol intake of more than the six beers a day reported earlier. The adjustment of severity ratings as treatment proceeds and the usefulness of tracking impairment severity as one way of measuring and articulating the patient's progress in treatment are addressed in Chapter 9.

Conclusion

The assignment of a severity rating to each of the impairments is a convenient, shorthand method for documenting and graphically summarizing the seriousness of the patient's condition. When we refer to communications with external reviewers, we are simultaneously proposing that the PIP (impairments and their severities) can be used to organize the treatment documentation in the medical record. It makes sense that the medical record should contain the information that managed care reviewers need to know, especially now, as computerized patient records become the norm over the next half-dozen years. Several large managed care organizations are already site-testing electronic information networks with their panel providers and facilities to expedite the case management process. This method of recording information is in the interest of the patient, the practitioner, and the reviewer. More is said about treatment documentation in Chapters 9 and 10, wherein we offer a model that satisfies the multiple documentation requirements that mental healthcare practitioners and facilities are currently expected to meet.

For the present, when talking on the telephone with a reviewer about the seriousness of the patient's condition, we offer the PIP and describe each impairment's severity (i.e., imminently dangerous, severely incapacitating, destabilizing, or distressing); we then offer two or three patient behaviors or patient statements that corroborate that severity rating. This is the clinical information reviewers need to know to justify treatment.

During the initial contact with the reviewer, more information is usually requested from the practitioner (e.g., the goals and objectives, the treatment plan, and the estimated length of stay or duration of treatment). How the practitioner responds to these questions is the subject of the next two chapters.

Chapter 7

Treatment Goals and the Patient Objectives

"What are the goals and objectives?"

In this chapter, we review the confusion and inconsistency surrounding "goals" and "objectives" and suggest supporting the appropriateness of treatment with the expected patient outcomes. Patient objectives belong to and are met by the patient, not the practitioner. Outcome-focused patient objectives are determined for each impairment in the patient's profile. In more intensive treatment, one or more patient objectives will be designated as "target objectives"—objectives whose completion signals readiness for discharge to less service-intensive care. The treatment goal is reasonable "repair" of the "impair"ments, marking the end of treatment.

Justification for treatment and a treatment setting is accomplished by specifying the severities of the patient's impairments and the anticipated benefits (outcome) of their treatment. Describing the expectations for the patient's treatment is often the most elusive task for the mental health practitioner—and the most pivotal one for the case manager or reviewer. Intentions such as "patient will be less depressed" or "patient will express feelings more appropriately" are not enough. What is missing in these statements is the rest of the sentence—that is, "patient will be less depressed as evidenced by. . . . " The patient impairment profile (PIP) coaxes the practitioner to establish meaningful and specific behavioral "patient objectives" that will substantiate appropriateness based on outcome. The accreditation standards of the Joint Commission on Accreditation of Healthcare Organizations and recently released Medicare documentation guidelines both require patient objectives and measurement of performance. Not surprisingly, when we surveyed the largest nationally based managed mental healthcare organizations, we learned that each review organization has basically the same information needs also.

The PIP-based documentation used and described in this book meets these data requirements. The PIP is, in fact, an information model well suited for automation. As healthcare makes the transition to automated data management and electronic communication networks, much of the telephone case management and paper chase that practitioners now experience will cease. Nonetheless, all the requirements for meaningful treatment data will continue. The practitioner will comply with either a computer or a ballpoint pen. (More is said about the PIP information model and computerized medical records and communication networks in Chapter 10.)

Documentation Requirements for Goals and Objectives

Clinical records are intended to document the course of patient treatment from intake through discharge and follow-up. During the intake process, the presenting complaints, history of the present illness, medical history, and family and social histories are obtained; a mental status examination is performed; and the results of a DSM-IV (American Psychiatric Association 1994) multiaxial evaluation are recorded. We recommend including the PIP, which clearly conveys the reasons for the treatment (impairments) and their severities. For patients requiring treatment in an accredited hospital or residential facility, data concerning physical and psychological status (including life-threatening problems, as well as emotional and behavioral functioning) and social functioning compose the initial assessment and provide the individualized information necessary to develop a preliminary treatment plan.

Following the initial assessment and identification of the patient's needs, the clinician and appropriate members of the treatment team have the responsibility to perform any further assessments deemed appropriate. Such assessments might be related to nutritional, physical, vocational, educational, recreational, developmental, legal, or discharge planning needs or to physical or psychological diagnostic testing. The team must develop a written, comprehensive, and appropriate individualized treatment plan, incorporating and prioritizing all pertinent assessment information. Both ongoing and specified reassessment by the treatment team is performed to review the patient's status in response to treatment and update the treatment plan. The terms *initial* or *intake assessment, preliminary treatment plan, further assessment, reassessment,* and *individualized treatment plan* are specific references in the 1995 Mental Health Manual (MHM) (Joint Commission on Accreditation of Healthcare Organizations 1994). The MHM contains detailed standards of care for organizations providing mental health services, substance abuse services, and services for mentally retarded and developmentally disabled persons. The patient evaluation process, the type of detailed information that composes the various assessments and treatment plan, and some time frames for completion are spelled out in the MHM.

A particular PIP addresses the assessment requirements described in the 1995 MHM in that it summarily specifies the patient's identified and prioritized emotional, behavioral, physical, social, educational, and, when appropriate, legal, vocational, and nutritional needs (the impairments). Note that there is no requirement for a problem list. In fact, the term is not even mentioned in federal guidelines or the MHM. The PIP specifies all the patient's needs that require, and can benefit from, treatment. It also clarifies which impairments, based on their severity rating, require more intensive care.

It is axiomatic that treatment plans include "goals" and "objectives." Yet, an informal review of hundreds of individual practitioner and multidisciplinary treatment plans reveals a conspicuous absence of congruence in the understanding and use of these two terms. At times they appear to be interchangeable or combined together (e.g., "resolution of marital conflict"); at other times they are descriptors of endpoints for the patient to meet (e.g., "improved communication with spouse"); and, not infrequently, they are confused with practitioner interventions (e.g., "teach active listening skills").

The 1995 MHM offers clarification on this point. Standard TX.1.6 requires that the treatment plan contain "specific goals that the patient must achieve to attain, maintain, and/or reestablish emotional and/or physical health as well as maximum growth and adaptive capabilities." Note the emphasis on the fact that the goals are the patient's, not the practitioner's. Standards TX.1.7–1.7.2 require that the treatment plan state "specific objectives relating to goals identified in the assessment process," that the "objectives are expressed in behavioral terms that provide measurable indices of progress," and that "[for] each objective, a projected date of achievement is specified." The specific objectives are also the patient's objectives, not the practitioner's. The clarity of terms offered by the MHM, however, becomes muddied when juxtaposed with federal guidelines and individual state regulations with which practitioners must also comply.

Medicare guidelines call for both "long-range and short-range goals" but do not define those terms (Federal Register 1984, pp. 315–316). The distinction between the long-range and short-range goals of the federal guidelines is, we feel, a confusing and difficult one to make. Short-range goals appear to be guideposts representing intermediate time spans during care. A series of short-range goals, when met, should achieve a final, accomplishable, desirable result. The last short-range goal might well be the final one and would have been called the long-range goal if set at the beginning of the series. Short-range goals may be useful ongoing clinical tools, but only a long-range goal carries the connotation of outcome for an episode of care (R. L. Grant 1981). The MHM does not distinguish between long-range and short-range treatment goals.

If this were not bewildering enough, some states, such as Colorado, also require that the treatment plan contain "goals that are measurable and have identified target dates for their completion" (Colorado Department of Institutions 1977, p. 27). A *goal* in Colorado very closely approximates an *objective* for the Joint Commission. The term *measurable* carries the explicit need for some form of quantification—a task for which most mental healthcare practitioners have never been adequately trained. In addition, which goals are to be measured? The short-range goals? The long-range goals? Both? The 1995 MHM implies that achievement of goals occurs when the patient has "attain[ed] . . . maximum growth and adaptive capabilities" (Standard TX.1.6)—that is, the completion of treatment. Actual achievement dates are assigned only to the patient's measurable objectives.

In late 1994, the long-awaited Health Care Financing Administration/American Medical Association medical documentation guidelines for evaluation and management procedures were released (American Medical Association 1994). Medicare plans to provide practitioners and claims reviewers with this "advice" about preparing or reviewing documentation for these evaluation and management inpatient, outpatient, and consultation services. What sort of documentation, according to Medicare, can payers request?

> Payers may request information to validate:
>
> - the site of service;
> - *the medical necessity and appropriateness of the diagnostic and/or therapeutic services provided* [emphasis added]; and/or
> - that services provided have been accurately reported. (Transamerica Occidental Life 1994, p. 2)

Treatment Goals

When the PIP is used for creating a treatment plan, a *treatment goal* is defined as the amelioration or "repair" of an impairment or the anticipated reduction in the severity rating of an impairment in the PIP. Goal achievement as stated in the 1995 MHM is expressed in the language of impairments by the repair of the impairment profile: the patient is returned to maximum wellness ("maximum growth and adaptive capabilities" [Standard TX.1.6]). Of course, the optimal goal for a patient is the absence of any impairment (technically this is a severity rating of 0).

At the time of assessment, we tend to set our sights high and anticipate that the patient's impairments can be eliminated.

Treatment goal: The repair of an impairment or reduction in severity of an impairment to an endpoint or maintenance level.

However, a patient's limitations or deficiencies may make the attainment of such a goal not possible. The treatment goal for each impairment must then be reevaluated and adjusted, when necessary, to reasonably achievable levels. For example, some patients with the impairment of Delusions (Paranoid) may never be free from persecutory or jealous delusional beliefs. However, reducing the disabling intensity of those beliefs with the proper medication might be an achievable goal.

There are two distinct clinical situations, however, when the treatment goal is not the repair of the impairment (severity 0) and the achievement of the treatment goal does not signify the completion of treatment. The treatment goals in these two instances are referred to as *maintenance goals* and *interim goals,* respectively.

Maintenance Goals

Patients who will require long-term or indefinite mental health treatment for an impairment to prevent a relapse (i.e., an increase in the impairment's severity rating) will carry a "maintenance goal." For example, a patient with an impairment of Delusions (Paranoid)—severity 1—may be able to manage activities of daily living and self-care adequately. If the Delusions exacerbate to severity 3, for example, and the patient requires hospitalization, the hospital treatment goal for the Delusions would be "severity rating for Delusions will be (maintenance) 1"—a maintenance goal.

Interim Goals

Patients who are receiving more costly treatment (e.g., inpatient care), and who on discharge will continue to receive treatment services, are not expected to be free of all impairments at the time of their first transition. Discharge to less intensive treatment is justified by a reduction in the severity of the patient's impairment. In this case, the impairment severity rating anticipated for that impairment at the time of discharge (to a lower level of care) becomes an "interim goal." Interim goals are provided for both case examples at the end of the chapter.

Patient Objectives

In a vertically integrated system of mental health services, multiple levels of care are available (e.g., intensive inpatient care, partial hospitalization, day treatment services, intensive outpatient treatment, medication management). Except when the patient is receiving the least intensive treatment (on completion of which the patient is supposed to be well), the designated patient objectives are to be met at the time of completion of a particular intensity of treatment. From that point, the patient moves on to a less intensive treatment with new patient objectives established for each impairment specific for that level. The estimated length of time it will take for the patient to meet these objectives is the answer to the reviewer's question regarding the length of stay or duration of treatment.

During the initial telephone contact with an outside reviewer, predictable questions are typically asked (although never in the same order) regarding the treatment plan, the goals and objectives, and the estimated length of treatment. Using the impairment model, we respond by providing the reviewer with specific patient objectives selected for each impairment in the profile. A patient objective is an anticipated statement or behavior by the patient that demonstrates progress toward repair of an impairment. Every patient objective must be "reasonable"—that is, each one accommodates the realities of the patient's strengths and limitations, the presence of other (comorbid) impairments, and the availability of resources to pay for the proposed treatment. We indicate that we expect these patient objectives to be met by completion of the particular intensity of treatment we are recommending. We also state which of these patient objectives are the target objectives and then explain that achieving the target objectives will signal the patient's readiness for discharge from that particular treatment intensity or setting. Achievement of the target objectives for the impairments is the behavioral evidence for the anticipated reduction in severity of the patient's impairments—the treatment goals.

Patient objective: An anticipated patient statement or behavior that demonstrates progress toward repair of an impairment.

Target objective: An anticipated patient statement or behavior that signals "discharge" to less service-intensive treatment.

In Appendix C, we provide the practitioner with a reference list of patient objectives for the (potentially) critical impairments. These objectives are divided into the "patient will verbalize" and "patient will demonstrate" categories. Achievement of a patient objective is evidenced by the say/do behavior of the patient. Wherever possible, the Appendix orders the patient objectives by increasing complexity or difficulty for the patient. Appendix C does not distinguish the target objectives because making that determination is an individualized clinical decision between the practitioner and the patient.

✻ *A note of caution: The patient objectives provided in Appendix C for these impairments are not definitive sets of criteria, all of which must be met by the patient, nor are they the only patient objectives suitable for a patient's impairments. The practitioner and patient may decide that other say/do behaviors will determine whether treatment is effective and the patient is satisfied.*

Case Examples

In the two clinical vignettes presented here, we include the initial patient objectives determined for both patients' impairments at the time of the initial assessment. In the case of Bob D., his initial impairment profile changed significantly by the third day of hospitalization when the team treatment plan was written. The integration of the assessments and observational data in this case required that the profile be updated to reflect accurately the evolving dynamic understanding of the case. Bob's patient objectives would be reevaluated and changed as well. (The consensually agreed-on PIP that resulted and the revised patient objectives are included in the description of the development of Bob's multidisciplinary treatment plan in Chapter 9.)

Target objectives for both patients' critical impairments (those rated severity 3 or 4) are expected to be met by the time of the patients' discharge from the acute treatment setting. Completing the patient objectives is the behavioral evidence for reaching the interim goals. The objectives for the noncritical impairments, when met, will mark the end of treatment. The patient objectives for the noncritical impairments are not the primary indicators of progress for the acute care (i.e., hospitalization) that both of these patients received. However, the presence of patient objectives for the noncritical impairments is significant because these impairments often may impact the treatment of the critical ones and may explain why meeting the target objectives for the critical impairments is delayed.

The discharge plans for both patients included further treatment in the respective appropriate settings. For both Melanie W. and Bob D., interim goals (specific reductions in the severity ratings of their critical impairments) were identified. Melanie, on discharge from the hospital, would continue in a day treatment program along with weekly individual psychotherapy and weekly family therapy. Bob would require additional outpatient psychotherapy while adhering to his sobriety program. Their readiness for discharge would hinge on their achieving the target objectives designated for each of them. Target objectives are identified on both patients' treatment plans with an asterisk (*).

Case 1: Melanie W.

Patient Impairment Profile Patient: Melanie W.

	Severity Rating	
Impairment	2/9	Interim Goal
1. Suicidal Thought/Behavior	4	2
2. Dysphoric Mood	4	3
3. Concomitant Medical Condition (juvenile-type diabetes mellitus)	4	2
4. Inadequate Healthcare Skills	2	—
5. Family Dysfunction	2	—
6. Truancy	2	—

Patient Objectives

(To Be Met by Discharge: 3/2/95)
(* = Target Objective)

Suicidal Thought/Behavior

Patient will verbalize:

• Plans to harm oneself rather than act on them.
• The precipitants for Suicidal Thought/Behavior.
• Alternative actions to be taken when feeling suicidal.
• Reasons for living.
* Warning signs that Suicidal Thought/Behavior is exacerbating.
* A plan of action to be taken should Suicidal Thought/Behavior exacerbate.

Patient will demonstrate:

• Participation in a prescribed treatment program.
• Commitment to a behavioral contract not to harm oneself.
* Elimination of Suicidal Thought/Behavior.
* A completed self-care (discharge) plan, including steps to be taken should Suicidal Thought/Behavior return or exacerbate.

Dysphoric Mood

Patient will verbalize:

• Awareness of severe mood changes when they occur.
• Awareness of the precipitating factors for negative mood changes.
• Statements that are positive and hopeful rather than negative and self-deprecating.
* Warning signs that the Dysphoric Mood is exacerbating.
* A plan of action to be taken should the Dysphoric Mood exacerbate.

Patient will demonstrate:

• Participation in a prescribed treatment program.
• Increased self-initiated and self-directed activities.
• Increased integrating behaviors with others.
* Reduction in the Dysphoric Mood as evidenced by a 50% decrease in the Hamilton Rating Scale for Depression (rated at the initiation of treatment) and/or a 50% improvement in the Coopersmith Self-Esteem Inventory.
* A completed self-care (discharge) plan, including steps to be taken should the Dysphoric Mood return or exacerbate.

Concomitant Medical Condition (juvenile-type diabetes mellitus)

Patient will verbalize:

- Thoughts and feelings regarding the medical condition.
- * Acceptance of responsibility for management of the medical condition.
- * Warning signs that the medical condition is exacerbating.
- * A plan of action to be taken should the medical condition exacerbate.

Patient will demonstrate:

- Adherence to the treatment regimen for the medical condition (e.g., self-initiated medication compliance, self-selected appropriate diet).
- * A self-care worksheet that describes the medical condition, its etiology, prognosis, treatment regimen, and potential future complications.
- * Adequate management of the medical condition.

Patient Objectives

(To Be Met by the End of Treatment: 7/10/95)

Inadequate Healthcare Skills

Patient will verbalize:

- Acceptance of responsibility for the Inadequate Healthcare Skills.
- Warning signs that the healthcare skills are deteriorating.
- A plan of action to be taken should healthcare skills deteriorate.

Patient will demonstrate:

- Adherence to the treatment program for the Inadequate Healthcare Skills.
- A self-care worksheet that describes the specific healthcare issues needing to be addressed.
- The ability to bathe, brush teeth, comb hair, and wear clean clothes daily.
- The ability to select nutritious foods from the four food groups at mealtime.
- Adequate healthcare skills.

Family Dysfunction

Patient will verbalize:

- Understanding of each family member's role in the Family Dysfunction.

- A plan for modifying the patient's own role within the family.
- The warning signs that the family is again becoming dysfunctional.
- A contingency plan of action to be taken should the Family Dysfunction increase.

Patient will demonstrate:

- Discussion with family members regarding each other's dysfunctional roles.
- A written clarification of the "nonnegotiables" for each family member.
- A written family contract that specifies the plans for change in the Family Dysfunction and the actions to be taken when significant disagreement occurs.
- Adherence to a written family contract.
- Elimination of distressing Family Dysfunction.

Truancy

Patient will verbalize:

- The precipitants for truant behaviors.
- Acceptance of responsibility for the Truancy.
- An alternative plan of action to take when thoughts to be truant occur.

Patient will demonstrate:

- A written paper that identifies the precipitating factors and the adverse consequences of being truant.
- Successful negotiation of a contract with the family regarding the consequences of continued Truancy.
- Meeting with an educator/counselor to develop a plan/contract for repairing the specific educational deficits resulting from Truancy.
- Adherence to the family contract regarding school/work attendance.
- Elimination of Truancy.

Melanie's impairments remained the same throughout her hospitalization. In the absence of unanticipated changes in the course of her treatment, the patient objectives and the target objectives were also to remain unchanged.

Case 2: Bob D.

Patient Impairment Profile **Patient: Bob D.**

Impairment	Severity Rating 9/1	Interim Goal
1. Delusions (Nonparanoid)	**4**	**2**
2. Substance Abuse (Alcohol)	**4**	**2**
3. Tantrums	**2**	**—**

Patient Objectives

(To Be Met by Discharge: 9/22/95)

(* = Target Objective)

Delusions (Nonparanoid)

Patient will verbalize:

- Awareness of the presence of delusional thinking.
- Responsibility for the presence of the Delusions.
- The precipitants for the delusional thinking.

* A plan of action to be taken should the Delusions exacerbate.

Patient will demonstrate:

- Adherence to the medical treatment of the Delusions.

* Absence of Delusions for 72 hours.

- Adequate management of the Delusions.

* A completed self-care (discharge) plan, including steps to be taken should the Delusions return or exacerbate.

Substance Abuse

Patient will verbalize:

- Acceptance of personal responsibility for the Substance Abuse.
- The precipitants for past Substance Abuse.
- The potential hazards of substance substitution.
- The warning signs that the urge to abuse is returning.

* A contingency plan of action to be taken should urge to abuse persist.

* A plan of action to be taken should a relapse occur.

Patient will demonstrate:

- Adherence to a medication/treatment program for the Substance Abuse.
- Completion of "Step One," which satisfactorily records the adverse impact of the Substance Abuse on the patient's and others' lives.
- A three- to five-page paper that addresses Substance Abuse as a disease, the problems of substance substitution, the relapse indicators, and relapse avoidance techniques.
- Obtaining a 12-step program sponsor.

* Abstinence from substances of abuse as evidenced by negative, random urine drug screenings.

Patient Objectives

(To Be Met by the End of Treatment: 12/11/95)

Tantrums

Patient will verbalize:

- Adverse consequences of the Tantrums.
- Alternative behaviors to the Tantrums.
- Acceptance of personal responsibility for the precipitants of the Tantrums (e.g., poor frustration tolerance).
- Feelings of anger instead of demonstrating the anger through Tantrums.

Patient will demonstrate:

- Adherence to the treatment program for the Tantrums.
- Ability to interrupt Tantrums before they occur.
- Elimination of Tantrums.

Conclusion

Both of these patients' hospital stays were subject to concurrent review that monitored the clinical necessity and appropriateness of further inpatient treatment. The critical impairments' severities and the reasonable patient objectives defined for the impairments become a readily inferred clinical rationale for treatment. The patient's progress toward meeting these objectives demonstrates that the treatment is working and that the patient is improving, even though the severity of a particular impairment may not have yet changed or may have dropped only one rating. Balancing "the patient is getting better" with "the patient is still very sick" is a much less precarious task with such measurable information about the patient. Statements such as "Melanie is smiling more and attending her activities without prompting" communicate the progress and effectiveness of her treatment. Evidence that the patient is still at risk—for example, "Melanie returned to her room in tears after she exploded in a family session with her mother and father; she then told a nurse that 'I was right all along. Nothing's ever going to change! Things are hopeless!'"—substantiates the necessity for continued intensive treatment, with a corresponding severity rating of 4.

Just as the impairments direct the determination of severity ratings, and the PIP drives the designation of specific patient objectives, the patient objectives, in turn, organize the selection of appropriate treatment interventions. This portion of the treatment plan does belong to the practitioner and not the patient. How the practitioner's interventions link to the impairments, severities, and patient objectives is the subject of Chapter 8.

Chapter 8

Practitioner Interventions and the Treatment Plan

"How are you planning to treat the patient?"

In this chapter, we describe how treatment modalities and specific practitioner interventions are determined by the patient objectives and treatment goals. A sequence of interventions implemented over time ought to parallel a decrease in impairment severity and an improvement in the patient. Practitioner interventions for individual psychotherapy are defined and distinguished from the more comprehensive "treatment plan." With the inclusion of treatment modalities (and practitioner interventions), the clinical vignettes demonstrate completed treatment plans. A model for a standardized treatment documentation format in mental health is presented.

Managed care review has taught mental health practitioners to anticipate questions about *goals, objectives, interventions,* and *treatment plans.* These familiar and ubiquitous terms occur in some combination in virtually all mental health patient records; one or more of them appear in most managed care companies' outpatient treatment reports, and these same terms often structure the telephone-based managed care review process as well. To the detriment of both the practitioner and the case manager, however, there are no universally accepted or gold standard definitions for these words. In this chapter, we examine and define practitioner interventions—the final component of the treatment plan—and describe the context for their links to both the patient objectives/treatment goals and the impairment severity rating. The necessity for a standardized method of treatment documentation is also addressed as an urgent concern for the mental health profession.

Practitioner Interventions

Treatment Modalities and Practitioner Interventions

From the vantage point of reimbursement for treatment services, mental healthcare is unique because a number of differently trained clinicians who also represent different disciplines (e.g., psychiatry, psychology, and social work) provide the same treatment modality and implement similar, if not identical, interventions. We define a *treatment modality* as a group or sequence of practitioner interventions employed as part of a therapeutic clinical service (e.g., individual psychotherapy). A *practitioner intervention* is an action taken by a trained mental health professional to modify, resolve, or stabilize the patient's impairments (e.g., "clarify the reason for a missed therapy appointment"). Although the difference in patient outcome as a result of this phenomenon remains an interesting, and as yet unanswered, question, several disciplines may bill for the same treatment service (e.g., individual psychotherapy, 45–50 minutes), employing the same Current Procedural Terminology (CPT) code (American Medical Association 1994). Even though practitioners from various disciplines are often reimbursed at different set rates, all providers may be subject to the same managed care review process.

Additionally, a single practitioner may provide more than one treatment modality (e.g., individual psychotherapy and biofeedback) and bill for these services separately using the appropriate codes. Each treatment modality may be individually reviewed for clinical necessity and appropriateness. More service-intensive treatment proposals often specify more than one treatment modality. In this case, different practitioners (e.g., a psychiatrist and a psychologist) may provide the different treatment modalities. For example, one may conduct conjoint therapy, while another practitioner implements a behavior modification program. In a hospital setting, the patient usually receives a number of treatment modalities: nursing services, individual psychotherapy, and some combination of other modalities such as family therapy, biofeedback, assertion training, dietary counseling, and so on. For these reasons, we recommend that practitioners sort and document their treatment interventions by treatment modality (e.g., family therapy) rather than by practitioner (e.g., psychologist) or by the practitioner's clinical discipline (e.g., social services).

We do not recommend that practitioners specify other modalities they may use later on; this applies to the interventions employed within a modality as well. Interventions planned for use later in treatment (e.g., mobilizing a patient's anger) should not be in the treatment plan until they are implemented. Similar to the disadvantage incurred with the "stuffed" problem list, stuffing the treatment plan with interventions is another case where "more is less." This makes clinical sense because, until all assessment data and the patient's response to initial treatment interventions are evaluated, it may not be clear, for example, whether a new patient found to be hallucinating is experiencing an exacerbation of a schizophrenic disorder or phencyclidine intoxication. The first interventions may well be the same (e.g., assessment of the patient, determination of a treatment setting, and, perhaps, initiating medication). However, with additional information, the treatment modalities or specific practitioner interventions subsequently selected for resolving the Hallucinations impairment may be very different, depending on the etiology.

* *Note to the practitioner:* *Some treatment modalities and some interventions may not be suitable or appropriate for a particular impairment, a particular impairment severity, or certain combinations of impairments. There are some impairments for which some treatment modalities and interventions may even be contraindicated. Practitioner interventions and*

treatment modalities are "necessary and appropriate" when there is reason to expect that the patient will improve as a result of them.

The interventions a practitioner plans to implement first or the interventions that are likely first to result in demonstrable patient progress are initially specified in the treatment plan. As treatment proceeds over time, an intervention may be 1) carried over unchanged; 2) completed, having served its intended purpose; 3) deleted as no longer appropriate; or 4) modified to suit a particular patient or need; additional interventions may be added. An intervention to be changed ought to remain on the treatment plan (set apart, for example, by running a dashed line through it), and the decision regarding why should be noted and dated in parentheses.

Practitioner Interventions and Patient Outcome

An obvious aspect of healthcare quality is the effectiveness of the treatment. Patient outcome is currently the most valid measure of clinical effectiveness of the practitioner interventions used—as well as a measure of performance for the clinical competence of the practitioner providing them. Patient outcome is a buzz phrase receiving a flurry of notoriety since being heralded by review organizations as impetus for the "fourth generation" of managed care review: *managed outcome.* The three previous generations have been described elsewhere as 1) *managed benefit reduction,* which restricted patient access to mental health services (beginning in the late 1970s); 2) *managed utilization,* a system that featured discounted fee-for-service networks controlled through utilization review; and, more recently, 3) *managed quality* through utilization management with an emphasis on determining the quality of the provider network (Geraty 1994).

Patient outcome data are now being collected by most managed care organizations. This information is currently derived from either 1) direct measurement of some aspect of patient functioning, using either practitioner- or patient-rated scales, or 2) patient satisfaction questionnaires. Examples of the former include the Brief Symptom Checklist and Integra System's Compass. The Quality of Life Inventory (QOLI), offered by National Computer Systems; PsychSentinel; the Health Status Questionnaire (HSQ); and the Rand Corporation Complaint of Depression (COD) telephone survey are examples of patient satisfaction inventories. One large nationally based managed care organization for mental health intends to use both types.

As is explained later in this chapter and in Chapter 10, the numerous and idiosyncratic documentation formats currently in use for recording mental healthcare treatment do not provide uniform data sets for meaningful outcomes research, intervention and practitioner profiling, and ultimately performance improvement. The availability of such data will have enormous implications for the future of mental healthcare delivery. The entire healthcare industry is being compelled to contend with accelerating demands for outcome data and standardized practice guidelines, and this consumer-driven requirement is most likely nonnegotiable. Unlike the exception made when diagnosis-related groups (DRGs) were implemented, the mental health and substance abuse specialties will not be exempt from this new imperative.

The result of a practitioner's interventions is an outcome. We "translated" the patient objectives (measures of patient outcome) into discrete quantifiable say/do patient behaviors to link them to practitioner interventions and actual patient outcomes. (The links between the impairments, the severity ratings, and the patient objectives are identified in Chapters 5, 6, and 7.) To identify correlations between different patients, different treatments, and different outcomes, common language links must be established to connect these aspects of patient care. The real value of the impairment terminology in the documentation format recommended in these chapters is its "power" to organize the abstract and often elusive narrative text of mental health treatment into data suitable for aggregation and multifunctional analysis. With healthcare on the brink of implementing computerized medical records, the patient impairment profile (PIP) method prepares mental health treatment information for sophisticated computer-assisted data analysis and for advanced electronic data information systems and networks.

To initiate clinical research on the effectiveness of interventions for repairing various impairments and different commonly occurring impairment aggregates, we have defined 12 categories of interventions. These are generic categories that summarize and condense the multitude of various therapeutic interventions mental health professionals are trained to provide. Although these categories are preliminary and perhaps arbitrary, we have nevertheless concluded that mental health practitioners certainly do the following:

1. *Assess* (and diagnose).
2. *Specify* treatment.
3. *Educate* patients and significant others.

4. *Validate* patients' thoughts and feelings.
5. *Suggest* ideas for patients to explore.
6. *Encourage* actions for patients to consider.
7. *Manipulate* patients' thoughts/actions (e.g., behavior modification).
8. *Confront* patients.
9. *Medicate* patients for symptom relief.
10. *Mobilize* affect connected to experiences and conflicts.
11. *Clarify* and *interpret* dynamics of symptoms.
12. *Discharge/terminate* patients from treatment.

These categories are used to identify the practitioner's interventions employed in the treatment modality of individual psychotherapy for the two case examples (Melanie W. and Bob D.) at the end of this chapter. With the identification of the therapeutic modalities and corresponding interventions planned for them, the treatment plans for both Melanie and Bob are now complete. Interventions and treatment modalities alone should not be confused with or considered the same as the treatment plan.

The Patient Treatment Plan

Lexical Land Mines

The "treatment plan" is familiar mental health jargon in use at least since accreditation and licensing agencies mandated its presence in patient records. A variety of definitions and assumptions as to what *is* a treatment plan exists in health standards references, treatment guidelines, and in the mental health literature. As a consequence, it is not unusual for the practitioner to be asked the following questions by four different reviewers on any given day:

- What is your treatment plan?
- What is the patient's treatment plan?
- What are the patient's goals and objectives?
- What are your goals?

While providing consultation to a number of providers who were appealing reimbursement denial decisions from several different managed care entities, we uncovered an astonishing fact about these commonplace terms: consensus about the definition and intended use of these treatment catchwords is conspicuously absent. When we tried to obtain some clarification by asking for definitions of these terms, none of the practitioners or any of the managed care reviewers gave the same answers. Even different reviewers within one managed care organization had different conceptions about these terms. Nobody could agree on the "correct" answer to questions such as

- Are the "goals" the practitioner's goals, the patient's goals, or the treatment goals?
- What is the difference between a "goal" and an "objective"?
- Whose "treatment plan" are we reviewing: the practitioner's plan or the patient's plan?

The more practitioners and managed care reviewers we asked about these stock phrases, the more numerous and varied were the answers. Yet, access to treatment for the patients hinged on the practitioners' response to questions using this very vocabulary. The providers and reviewers were walking over what we refer to as "lexical land mines" because, when detonated, meaningful communication about patients' (proposed) treatment is invariably sabotaged.

The Goal-Objective-Intervention (G-O-I) Survey

We have researched and substantiated this unexpected finding by conducting an informal survey of 156 licensed clinical mental health professional and managed care reviewers. Each participant was provided with a one-page list of 20 statements (the Goal-Objective-Intervention [G-O-I] Survey) and then instructed to decide (placing a check mark in the appropriate column) whether each statement represents 1) a goal (G), 2) an objective (O), or 3) an intervention (I). All the participants had more than 2 years' clinical experience and had participated in at least six care-managed patients' reviews. Of the participants, 133 (85%) were either Ph.D. clinical psychologists (39%) or M.D. psychiatrists (46%) engaged in at least half-time clinical practice. The remainder of the participants (15%) were managed care reviewers who by training were either licensed clinical social workers (8%), Ph.D. clinical psychologists (4%), or M.D. psychiatrists (3%). The statements in the questionnaire were not composed by us. In fact, they were culled from the treatment records we had been reviewing for appeal following denials for further authorized care. The first five statements from the survey are as follows:

1. Alleviate the depressed mood.
2. Develop assertiveness skills.
3. Resolve marital conflicts.
4. Implement a "no-suicide" contract.
5. Establish a therapeutic alliance.

Of the 20 statements used in this survey, 7 were, in fact, treatment goals; 7 were patient objectives; and 6 were interventions. (Answers to the above five statements are given and provided with explanations toward the end of this chapter.) Interestingly, the responses on each individual survey were fairly evenly distributed among goals, objectives, and interventions. When the results were aggregated, however, the group as a whole was divided in more or less equal thirds on each individual statement. The tabulated results are shown in Table 8–1.

There was less than 70% consensus on any one statement (106 respondents correctly identified one statement as a goal), and each statement was always represented as a goal, an objective, and an intervention at least 12% of the time. Neither the practitioner group nor the reviewer group fared better or worse than the other.

More Lexical Land Mines

A comparison of the information requirements on different treatment report forms used by two review organizations illustrates how endemic this perpetual potential for miscommunication has become. The two companies' forms document the problem we notice repeatedly in telephone-based managed care reviews and denial appeals. (The data elements of

Table 8–1. Results of the G-O-I Survey (in percent)

	Goal	Objective	Intervention
1. Alleviate the depressed mood	68	19	13
2. Develop assertiveness skills	41	53	12
3. Resolve marital conflicts	28	52	20
4. Implement a "no-suicide" contract	38	24	38
5. Establish a therapeutic alliance	26	30	44

these two forms have been scrambled and modified to maintain anonymity of both organizations while still preserving the essence of the inconsistencies and contradictions.)

Company A requests its providers periodically to complete a one-page treatment information form that includes five sections:

- Section I: Patient's diagnosis
- Section II: Problems and symptoms
- Section III: Treatment plan
- Section IV: Goals and target dates
- Section V: Criteria for termination of treatment

Although practitioners are certainly experienced in addressing such issues as these, this form poses several vagaries worth detailing. Section II asks the practitioner to describe problems and symptoms. Is a "problem" different from a "symptom"? If so, what distinguishes a "Company A problem" from a "Company A symptom"?

Regarding Section III, treatment plan, there is no other space on the form for practitioners to specify their interventions; is the practitioner supposed to list them here? Is a "Company A treatment plan" in fact a "practitioner treatment plan" (interventions)? Or, does Company A's treatment plan mean something else? Section IV, goals and target dates, implies listing several "goals" with (probably?) different "target dates." Are these goals and target dates a series of accomplishments to be met in a sequence? Are they perhaps similar to what are more often referred to as "objectives"? Or, do "Company A goals" mark the completion of treatment? If one thinks that this is the case, how then are they different from what is requested in Section V, criteria for termination of treatment?

Company B asks its providers to complete and return a two-page form entitled "Treatment Plan/Goals." In addition to requesting standard identifying information (which is not included here), the form has six sections to be completed:

- Section I: Diagnosis (DSM-IV: all five axes)
- Section II: Current symptoms and functioning (describe progress for resolving these problems)
- Section III: Expected duration of treatment
- Section IV: Treatment objectives (in behavioral terms)
- Section V: Dates of service to date, medications
- Section VI: Names of family members/significant others in treatment

The title of the form is a potential land mine by its own right. Is a "Company B treatment plan" the same as a "Company B goal"? If so, which is the synonym for which? Or, are treatment plan and treatment goals *two* Company B terms to be addressed separately on the form? One never knows for sure because neither of the terms is used again. Unlike Company A, Company B clearly defines what it means by "current symptoms" in Section II. For Company B, symptoms are the same as "problems." Section IV requests "treatment objectives (in behavioral terms)." Are Company B's treatment objectives referring to the "treatment goals"—or the "plan"—or the "plan/goals"—used in the title of this form? On the other hand, if Company B's treatment objectives are benchmarks of patient progress, this information was asked for in Section II (describe progress for resolving these problems). Or, does "progress" refer to changes in the interventions? One might conclude this, given that the practitioner's interventions are not requested anywhere else (other than in Sections V and VI, which ask only for dates of service to date, medications, and names of family members/significant others in treatment).f one compares the terminology used by Company A's and Company B's outpatient treatment reports, it might appear that each company is requesting different information about the patient's treatment. Of course, Company A and Company B could also be seeking very similar information while using their own idiosyncratic definitions or intended meanings for these terms. Our conclusion based on extended discussion with the largest nationally based managed care corporations (and other insurers) is that Companies A and B—like the rest of their colleagues—have virtually the same treatment plan information requirements. However, in the absence of national managed care review standards for systematically obtaining and assessing this information, and without a standardized language (or terminology) and format for recording mental health treatment (from which the necessary data could possibly be retrieved), this information is requested in as many different ways as there are reviewers and review organizations.

We came to understand why practitioners experience such bewilderment, frustration, and irritation when engaged in managed care reviews. Discussions about the clinical necessity of a patient's treatment proposal are perilous indeed with so many lexical land mines of treatment terminology ready to explode. To assume a stability of reference and a seamless web of meaning for these words is to disregard Humpty Dumpty's admonition to Alice—and us—in *Through the Looking Glass*: "Words don't mean what you think they mean. Everything depends on who's doing the talking!"

We will not belabor these two forms further. Clearly, the mental health profession lacks consensual agreement about what these treatment terms mean. However, without a consensus of meaning, there can be no effective communication. If clinical care documentation fails to communicate the process of patient treatment, then efforts by its providers to justify the value of mental health services and demonstrate the effectiveness and competence of its providers will also fail.

A Proposed Treatment Plan Documentation Standard

A standardized method for mental health treatment documentation with a clear definition of its component parts is desperately needed. Today's mental health treatment plan can no longer function as a perfunctory requirement that is completed after the fact, often only in time for a clinical audit, and, at least historically, "referred back to" only when necessary.

In a managed care environment, "managing" the care means "concurrent monitoring" of the process and progress of a patient's treatment. For documentation to provide answers to the questions managed care reviewers are asking, the treatment plan record must be current and "alive." As the telephone-based managed care review method continues to become more cumbersome and less efficient for both reviewers and practitioners, it is inevitable that the written (or laser-printed) word, rather than a telephone, will provide the means to determine whether treatment services are necessary, appropriate, and effective (and hence eligible for reimbursement). We are reminded of another early Medicare professional standards review organization (PSRO) axiom that now has new relevance: "If it isn't documented in the patient's chart [or in the electronic record], then it didn't happen!"

Current treatment documentation must summarily address several aspects of the care at any point in time. These aspects include 1) a description of the patient's present condition (comparing it with the initial presentation), 2) evidence of progress the patient is making in treatment, and 3) the anticipated endpoints of the current phase of treatment. The treatment record is a status report on each of these concerns; it can no longer be out of date only to be revised at predetermined intervals. A timely clinical record identifies any and all changes in the patient's condition, whether positive or negative. Recording these and any other changes (e.g., adding interventions) automatically updates this clinical record of patient care. Documentation phraseology, such as "clinical status unchanged" and "continue same treatment plan," has no value in the managed care environment. The treatment record format we are describing is clearly about and for the patient—not the practitioner. This is why we refer to the treatment plan as the *patient treatment plan.*

Adhering to treatment documentation standards can be perplexing when the terminology used is variable and inconsistent. Federal guidelines describe a "multidisciplinary" treatment plan, seeming to emphasize the role of the treatment team (Federal Register 1984), whereas the 1995 Mental Health Manual (MHM) (Joint Commission on Accreditation of Healthcare Organizations 1994) refers to an "individualized" treatment plan, seeming to focus on the patient. Federal guidelines describe the plan as "the prescribed treatment, treatment given, and long- and short-term goals" (Federal Register 1984, pp. 315–316); MHM Standard TX 1.8 requires the plan to state "specific goals" and "specific objectives," and specify "settings, services, or programs necessary to meet the individual's needs and goals." As is often the case, accreditation standards are again reshaping the treatment plan document—this time with the focus on the patient. Instead of practitioners being asked, "How are you managing the patient?" now the question becomes, "How is the patient managing?"

In the collaborative restorative effort between a practitioner and a patient that is called *treatment,* both participants contribute to the clinical record. The primary practitioner is responsible for providing the following information in a patient treatment plan:

- Assessment
- Diagnosis
- Interventions (or modalities)
- Discharge plan

We refer to the practitioner's contributions as the *operational component* of the treatment plan.

The ambiguous "ownership" of the diagnosis—is it the practitioner's or the patient's?—initiates the eventual confusion over a larger issue: whose treatment plan is it—the practitioner's or the patient's? The focus on diagnostic classification is distracting in that it may obscure the patient's predicaments and reported difficulties in life (impairments). Unfortunately, this fact is entrenched by an insurance industry that pays for a diagnosis, not for the patient's predicaments or difficulties. DSM-IV cautions, " . . . diagnosis is only the first step in a comprehensive evaluation. *To formulate an adequate treatment plan, the clinician will invariably require considerable additional information* about the person being evaluated beyond that required to make a DSM-IV diagnosis" (p. xxv, emphasis added).

The patient's contribution to the clinical record is the comparative information that convincingly communicates *change in the patient*—in thoughts and ideas, moods and emotions, and in behavior. This *process component* of the treatment plan is qualitative, behavior based, and discretely measurable in contrast to the practitioner's more abstract and synthesized operational component. The process component of the patient treatment plan includes

- Impairments
- Impairment severities
- Patient objectives (including target objectives)
- Treatment goals

In a patient treatment plan, the assessment, diagnosis, and discharge plan (the operational components) typically remain unchanged in a course of treatment. The interventions *may* change, for example, if they are no longer unnecessary or become inappropriate. Patient change (the process component) is, of course, anticipated and welcomed, and there is cause for concern when it is not in evidence. This process component and the operational component conjoin to form a comprehensive description of patient care. Therefore, we believe that a complete patient treatment plan contains and records over time any and all changes in the

- Assessment
- Diagnosis
- PIP (impairments may remain the same over the course of treatment; the severity ratings are expected to decrease over time)
- Patient objectives (although both treatment goals and patient objectives may remain the same, the incremental progress the patient is demonstrating toward achieving the objectives also must be documented)
- Treatment goals
- Practitioner interventions
- Discharge plan

Treatment Plan Terminology

The definitions for the elements of a patient treatment plan have been given in various sections of this book. They are recapitulated below for comparison, cross-reference, and convenience.

Assessment The systematic collection and analysis of the individual-specific data necessary to determine patient care needs, including at least the history, physical and mental status examinations, and any diagnostic tests or studies.

Diagnosis A decision regarding the nature of a mental disorder (using DSM-IV or ICD-9-CM nomenclature) based on an examination of symptoms.

Discharge plan A prescribed course of action to be implemented when the patient is released or dismissed from a treatment setting or treatment, based on assessment of the patient's status and need for continuing care.

Impairment A behavior-based descriptor of patient dysfunction.

Intervention An action taken by a trained mental health professional to modify, resolve, or stabilize the patient's impairments.

Patient impairment profile (PIP) The impairments that are prioritized as the focus of treatment and their respective severity ratings.

Patient objective An anticipated patient statement or behavior that demonstrates progress toward repair of an impairment.

Severity rating A description of the degree of 1) danger or risk to self or others or 2) compromised function due to an impairment (for mental health impairments).

Target objective An anticipated patient statement or behavior that signals "discharge" to less service-intensive treatment.

Treatment goal The repair of an impairment or reduction in severity of an impairment to an endpoint or maintenance level. The anticipated reduction in impairment severity may be an *interim goal* or a *maintenance goal*.

Treatment modality A group or sequence of practitioner interventions employed as part of a therapeutic clinical service.

Answers to the G-O-I Survey

Returning to the G-O-I Survey mentioned earlier in this chapter, the answers for the first five items and a brief rationale for each of them are as follows:

1. *Alleviate the depressed mood* is a treatment goal. Based on repairing the impairment of Dysphoric Mood, this is an endpoint of treatment.
2. *Develop assertiveness skills* is a patient objective. Although the practitioner may enhance the patient's skills in this area using several interventions, the patient is the one who acquires the skill (usually as a benchmark of progress toward resolving an impairment such as Marital/Relationship Dysfunction).
3. *Resolve marital conflicts* is a goal. This is based on repairing the Marital/Relationship Dysfunction impairment.
4. *Implement a "no-suicide" contract* is a patient objective. A practitioner may suggest, write, or even sign such a contract with a patient; however, adhering to the contract—implementing and using it to learn how to manage suicidal thoughts more adaptively—is a patient action (and benchmark of progress for repair of the Suicidal Thought/Behavior impairment).
5. *Establish a therapeutic alliance* is a patient objective. Although facilitating the development of a therapeutic or treatment alliance is a skill for which mental health professionals are specifically trained—a skill that includes conveying a nonjudgmental attitude, adapting a posture of support and acceptance, and so on—its establishment entirely hinges on the patient to demonstrate that this objective has occurred.

Case Examples

We return to the cases of Melanie W. and Bob D. and include the treatment modalities selected for these patients. In consideration of space, the generic interventions will be specified only for individual psychotherapy. Although we have previously cautioned practitioners to avoid stuffing the treatment plan with interventions, at the same time it is important that practitioners also be credited for their efforts. The more documented interventions that can be correlated with a favorable outcome, the larger the database will be to substantiate the clinical effectiveness of various interventions. An in-depth computer-assisted analysis of such data may reveal more subtle information about an intervention's effectiveness for 1) an impairment when it appears with certain other (comorbid) impairments or 2) different severities of the same impairment. All the while, of course, a database is also being aggregated for substantiating the clinical competence of the practitioner—as well as calling attention to the noteworthy benefit of mental health treatment in general.

Case 1: Melanie W.

Treatment Plan Patient: Melanie W.

Patient Impairment Profile

Impairment	Severity Rating 2/9	Interim Goal
1. Suicidal Thought/Behavior	4	2
2. Dysphoric Mood	4	3
3. Concomitant Medical Condition (juvenile-type diabetes mellitus)	4	2
4. Inadequate Healthcare Skills	2	—
5. Family Dysfunction	2	—
6. Truancy	2	—

Patient Objectives

See Chapter 7 for a complete list of Melanie W.'s patient objectives.

Practitioner Interventions

Suicidal Thought/Behavior

Individual psychotherapy:

- Assess the need for evaluation by specific support services: psychological testing, social services, activities therapy, psychodrama.
- Validate her stated reasons for the despondency.
- Confront the patient's suicidal behavior by attempting to establish a "no-suicide" contract.
- Clarify the dynamics of the patient's wishes to destroy herself.

Nursing:

Discharge planning services:

Group psychotherapy:

Dysphoric Mood

Individual psychotherapy:

- Clarify the nature of the Dysphoric Mood.

- Evaluate for antidepressant medication.
- Mobilize affect about the struggle with her mother's chronic depression.
- Suggest the patient explore the connections between the dysphoric episodes and the periods of increased somatic complaints.
- Educate the patient to differentiate and to label accurately more of her feeling states.

Nursing:

Group psychotherapy:

Recreational therapy:

Creative arts therapy:

Concomitant Medical Condition (juvenile-type diabetes mellitus)

Individual psychotherapy:

- Reinforce ("manipulate") with identifiable rewards the diligent and accurate monitoring of her blood and urine diabetes testing four times a day.
- Educate the patient regarding her misconceptions about juvenile-onset diabetes mellitus.
- Support expression of "secret fears" about the diabetes.

Nursing:

Group psychotherapy:

Nutritional and dietary counseling:

Inadequate Healthcare Skills

Individual psychotherapy:

- Confront the patient's specific areas of poor self-care.
- Clarify the reasons for the poor self-care.

Nursing:

Nutritional and dietary counseling:

Family Dysfunction

Individual psychotherapy:

- Suggest that the patient may have a role in the Family Dysfunction that needs to be identified and understood.
- Support the patient in verbalizing apprehensions about attending family therapy.

Family therapy:

Truancy

Individual psychotherapy:

- Suggest the patient determine and accurately verbalize the causes for being habitually truant.
- Confront her about the extent of education deficit as a result of the Truancy.
- Assess for presence of a possible learning disability.

Family therapy:

Education services:

Case 2: Bob D.

Treatment Plan — Patient: Bob D.

Patient Impairment Profile

Impairment	Severity Rating 9/1	Severity Rating Interim Goal
1. **Delusion**	4	0
2. **Substance Abuse (Alcohol)**	4	2
3. **Tantrums**	2	—

Patient Objectives

See Chapter 7 for a complete list of Bob D.'s patient objectives.

Practitioner Interventions

Delusions

Individual psychotherapy:

- Assess the etiology of the Delusions.
- Validate the patient's belief that the Delusions are real.
- Educate the patient about the nature of Delusions.
- Support the patient's attempts to distinguish what is real and what is not.

- Treat the Delusions with antipsychotic medication.
- Suggest that the patient comply with the medication plan to reduce misbeliefs that have resulted in unfortunate encounters with the law and family.

Nursing:

Substance Abuse (Alcohol)

Individual psychotherapy:

- Assess the patient for medical detoxification.
- Validate the intensity of the patient's fear that without alcohol he will totally lose control and possibly injure someone unintentionally.
- Suggest and educate the patient about the effectiveness of 12-step programs for alcohol abuse in conjunction with problem-focused psychotherapy.
- Educate the patient about alternatives to Substance Abuse for self-regulation of tension and anxiety.

Nursing:

Substance abuse counseling:

Group psychotherapy:

Family psychotherapy:

Nutritional and dietary counseling:

Recreation therapy:

Tantrums

Individual psychotherapy:

- Assess the patient for a Concomitant Medical Condition.
- Suggest that the patient focus and identify what the "triggers" might be for the Tantrums.
- Validate the patient's difficulty in tolerating even minimal frustration.
- Confront the patient about the real consequences of his unacceptable Tantrum behaviors.

Nursing:

Occupational therapy:

Family therapy:

Conclusion

The PIP (impairments with severity ratings), in tandem with the patient objectives, treatment goals, and practitioner interventions, constitutes the patient's treatment plan. This treatment plan model expediently organizes the patient's clinical record and simplifies the maintenance of a meaningful, current, and pertinent patient status report. We fully recognize that producing comprehensive patient treatment plans using the method described in this book is a time-consuming endeavor. However, when practitioners use this format, updating the treatment plan does become easier and quicker. Because the treatment plan is always a current summary of the course of the treatment, when the patient is ready for discharge, 90% of the discharge summary is already completed as well. Also, a treatment plan is already in place, at least in draft, if a patient resumes treatment after an interruption in the care. The effort spent in coordinating the initial patient treatment plan is an investment that pays well over time. A great deal of clinical information can be conveyed with a minimum of words once the treatment plan is in place.

Chapter 9

Patient Progress and Outcome

"How is the patient progressing?"

During the course of treatment, an up-to-date PIP-based treatment plan provides convincing evidence for justifying additional necessary care. In both individual and multidisciplinary treatment settings, updating the plan consists of a reevaluation of each impairment and severity and assessment of the patient's progress toward meeting each objective. Achieving patient objectives and reaching the goals of treatment notarize the effectiveness of the treatment and constitute a good outcome. Two case examples are included.

Obtaining authorization from reviewers for further treatment is probably the most challenging, and at times vexing, component of the review process. In our experience, when practitioners are able to articulate their clinical rationale for continuing care, using specific patient behaviors to describe both patient progress and clinical necessity for the care, this task becomes considerably easier. When requesting authorization for additional treatment, we restate the patient objectives agreed on in the original contact with the reviewer and provide a patient behavior that communicates the patient's progress toward meeting each objective and any adjustment of the severity ratings of the impairments in the patient impairment profile (PIP). We then offer supportive behavioral statements that substantiate how severely impaired the patient still may be. The balancing of behavioral statements that describe the patient's progress toward meeting objectives with behaviors that corroborate the current severity of the impairments provides the reviewer with the clinical rationale needed to make accurate decisions regarding the clinical necessity and appropriateness for continued treatment at a particular service intensity.

In many cases we have been able to substitute written summaries for the direct contact with reviewers and thereby significantly reduce time spent on the telephone. These reports are no more than an updated PIP, with adjusted severity ratings, patient objectives, and descriptors of the patient's behaviors that support both the current severity of each impairment and the patient's progress toward meeting the objectives. Additional detail regarding the process of the treatment (e.g., what specifically transpired in each of the treatment modalities) is usually not necessary.

We have found that most reviewers not only cooperate but, in fact, appreciate the time saved using this systematic format for providing patient care update information. There are three reasons for this generally favorable response. First, when the practitioner provides the reviewer a list of the patient objectives in the initial communication regarding clinical necessity of treatment services, an implicit agreement is established as to what specifically the patient needs to demonstrate before being treated in a less service-intensive setting. Second, because patient objectives are stated in behavioral terms, the patient's progress can be measured, scored, and tracked by degree of improvement. We provide numerical data when we can (e.g., a 50% improvement on the Beck Depression Inventory); otherwise, we offer a subjective estimate of the patient's progress toward meeting the patient objectives for each impairment (e.g., 25%, 50%, 75%, and 100% completed). We note that the practitioner's capability and accuracy in arriving at such percentages have not been an issue. Third, in the more intensive levels of service, where some review organizations monitor the patient's treatment and progress every 2 or 3 days, evidence of a patient's progress in meeting the objectives for an impairment can be seen before there is a reduction in the severity rating.

Even when an impairment continues to be severely incapacitating (severity 3) or imminently dangerous (severity 4), the patient's response to treatment interventions can still be demonstrated via the patient objectives. For example, after a week as an inpatient, Melanie W. (see case examples in preceding chapters) still required one-to-one supervision when testing her blood glucose and administering her insulin, and her Dysphoric Mood remained at severity 4. At the same time, she was making some progress toward her objectives as demonstrated by her improved grooming and personal hygiene.

The goal of treatment is, of course, reduction of the severity of the impairment. An impairment that is not dropping in severity with initial treatment interventions may be an "indicator" for more in-depth review. At the first level of more in-depth review, appropriate documentation and communication of the presence of the behavioral progress toward meeting specific patient objectives resolve the concern. If there is little or no demonstrable evidence of the patient's progress in meeting objectives, however, or if the patient is becoming worse, a second-level review may be performed, which in our experience examines any one or more of the following components of the treatment plan: 1) the patient objectives, 2) the treatment interventions, and 3) the PIP.

The patient objectives initially determined for an impairment may be unrealistic as the nature and extent of the patient's limitations and deficiencies are further revealed and understood in the early phases of treatment. Or, the patient objectives selected at the beginning of treatment may have become inappropriate or irrelevant for the patient over time. In the case of Bob D. (see case examples in preceding chapters), who presented initially with Delusions and Substance Abuse (Alcohol), the PIP changed significantly in the early course of his treatment, and, as a result, the patient objectives in the initial treatment plan were no longer pertinent. Lack of patient progress may also be calling attention to inappropriate or ineffectively implemented treatment interventions that would require the appropriate corrective action. At the same time, some treatment interventions (e.g., a course of electroconvulsive therapy or a trial on antidepressant medication) require a number of days before their effectiveness can be demonstrated.

Patient progress may also be impeded by the adhesiveness of an impairment (patient resistance)—perhaps due to the presence of other concomitant impairments that impede the patient's participation in the treatment milieu or in following individualized treatment recommendations. In the case of Melanie W., her ongoing difficulty with regulating the diabetes, her resulting frustration, and her increased sense of futility slowed the progress of treatment for her Dysphoric Mood. This information is helpful for reviewers who may be questioning, "Why isn't the patient getting any better?"

Multidisciplinary Treatment Planning

One of the requirements for exemption of psychiatric units from Medicare's system of prospective payment based on diagnosis-related groups (DRGs) is that each inpatient has a comprehensive treatment plan formulated by a multidisciplinary team (Federal Register 1984). The Joint Commission on Accreditation of Healthcare Organizations (1994), in the 1995 mental health manual (MHM), still requires "individualized and appropriate treatment plans" (TX.1) and refers to the provision of care "in a collaborative and interdisciplinary manner" (TX.1.2), with "staff participation from appropriate disciplines" (TX.1.3). Both Medicare and Joint Commission guidelines identify specific elements that must be in these plans. (These are detailed in Chapter 8 and are not repeated here.)

At its minimum operational level, the initial multidisciplinary treatment plan is a collation and summation of all the patient assessments performed by all providers of treatment services. The MHM requires the treatment plan to include, in addition to goals and objectives, a description of "the settings, services, or programs necessary to meet the individual's needs and goals" (TX.1.8). Although it is usually not possible for multidisciplinary treatment planning to take place at the time of admission, the MHM does expect that a designated treatment team develop the plan "within 72 hours following admission to any inpatient or residential treatment setting, or upon completion of the intake process for partial-hospitalization or outpatient treatment" (TX.1.1).

In today's inpatient settings, progress toward outcome usually has already begun to occur by the time the practitioner team convenes to develop the multidisciplinary treatment plan. A generic utilization review axiom states, "Discharge planning begins at the time of admission," to which we would add, "and so does the implementation of a treatment plan." The cost-conscious public, third-party payers, and managed care reviewers expect treatment to begin at the time of admission. Currently, multidisciplinary treatment plans (and updates) for psychiatric inpatient care usually do not reflect the treatment from time of admission. Fragments of the primary practitioner's initial treatment plan (including preliminary goals, objectives, and interventions) are often scattered among the patient history, the order sheets, and the progress notes. The documentation of the initial treatment efforts and the patient's progress during the customarily intensive first 3 days of treatment become eclipsed or overridden by the multidisciplinary treatment plan. Valuable information regarding the effectiveness of the practitioners' first interventions early in the illness, when the most dramatic changes in the PIP and the severity of the impairments are apt to occur, becomes difficult to find. Reviewers are generally sympathetic to the fact that a comprehensive assessment of the patient and the development of a meaningful multidisciplinary, individualized treatment plan may require 2 or 3 days to complete. However, after a patient has spent 3 days in an acute inpatient setting, reviewers will also want an update on the patient's progress.

Because the medical record is still the final source of information for quality and utilization monitoring, we have designed the documentation system to capture and to summarize graphically the patient's clinical course and progress from the initial assessment. In this context, an updated treatment plan also describes the process of the care and the progress of the patient evolving over time. We speculate that in the not-too-distant future, review organizations will put down the telephone and return to the treatment record—whether handwritten or computer generated—to determine clinical necessity and appropriateness of the treatment. The maxim "if it isn't documented, it didn't happen or it wasn't done" will still apply. Even now, a number of review organizations retrospectively review a percentage of medical records to confirm information received by telephone. When all clinical disciplines organize and discuss their understanding of the patient by impairments, severity ratings, patient objectives, and interventions, the result is an integrated and meaningful treatment plan and clinical record.

There is a current misconception that every practitioner who performs a treatment intervention for a patient must define goals and objectives for that patient. Although the idea of multidisciplinary treatment planning is that the team is working together, what we have observed is that when each treatment modality generates its own problem list, goals, and objectives for the patient, the result is "particle-ized" rather than "individualized" patient care.

In one patient's record that we reviewed, after totaling the objectives identified by the admitting psychiatrist, the psychiatric nurse, the social worker, the activities therapist, the substance abuse counselor, the nutritionist, the psychodramatist, and the art therapist, we discovered the patient had 43 different objectives to meet by the time of discharge! Obviously, this all makes no sense.

What does make sense to us is that at the time of initial assessment of the patient (Chapter 7), some one person—in a hospital setting, this is usually the admitting clinician; in an independent practice association, this is usually the clinician responsible for the triage or initial interview—identifies a preliminary PIP (impairments and severities), specifies probable and reasonable patient objectives for the impairments, indicates the initial treatment approach, and estimates the duration of treatment. (The estimated date of discharge [EDD], also referred to as the estimated length of stay [ELOS], is the date for completion of the target objectives.)

Other practitioners who may be involved in the patient's treatment can identify additional impairments during their assessments, or, if they believe that any of the preliminary impairments are not accurate, their findings are brought to the multidisciplinary treatment team meeting to be discussed when updating the PIP. What appears to be, for example, an impairment of profound Social Withdrawal may, with additional assessment information from team members, be due to the impairments of Hallucinations and Dysphoric Mood.

At the initial team meeting, the first question to be answered is which impairments remain and which are to be deleted, changed, or added to the PIP. Second, are there any changes in the severity rating of each impairment? The patient objectives identified in the initial treatment plan become the springboard for a discussion and decision by the treatment team as to which patient objectives are now the most appropriate for the patient's treatment plan. Each member of the treatment team can then ask, "Will any of the patient objectives be facilitated by my particular treatment modality?"

For example, the admitting clinician may include Dysphoric Mood on an initial PIP and identify one patient outcome objective for that impairment: "increased initiation of self-directed activities." After the team members consensually agree on the impairments and severities and the reasonable patient objectives, each practitioner can specify those treatment interventions that can facilitate accomplishment of the patient objectives. Continuing with the above example, the individual psychotherapist may utilize the intervention "clarify the nature and extent of the Dysphoric Mood" to help the patient identify the reasons for isolative behaviors. The activities therapist may initiate an interest inventory to discover new areas of curiosity and then support the patient in exploring them. Group therapy interventions, such as confronting the patient's irrational fears about new social situations, may facilitate accomplishment of this patient objective as well. All three disciplines will be using their own different treatment interventions, which are now integrated toward accomplishment of an objective and (ultimately) repair of the impairment (the treatment goal). In this way, the treatment plan becomes more than the sum of its parts.

Case Examples

The treatment plan should always be a current summary account of the team's treatment efforts and the patient's response to them. The two case examples, Melanie W. and Bob D., are sample formats that illustrate how the initial treatment plan, the progress of the patient, the practitioners' assessments, and their evolving understanding of the patient are recorded in the treatment plan.

Case 1: Melanie W.

Clinical Update

At the time of the first multidisciplinary team meeting, Melanie was still verbalizing active suicidal ideation daily. The day before, her second full day on the inpatient unit, she requested to be given a trial on "close observation" instead of the more scrutinizing one-to-one supervision. She was later found in the bathroom with a broken bobby pin scratching her wrist, which required two sutures. She insisted angrily that this was not a suicide attempt, however, "I was just pissed off at this place and all its stupid rules!" Melanie did acknowledge that she was "thinking about signing that no-suicide-attempt contract" but, as yet, was not ready to do so.

At the same time, the staff had noticed that she was now showering, brushing her hair, and dressing a bit more neatly. Melanie would get herself to some of the activities planned for her if she knew ahead of time they were "easy and fun." She was unable to concentrate in her classroom work for more than 5 minutes at a time. She did not complete any of her assignments and persisted in spending as much time in her room as the staff would allow. With the staff monitoring her during glucose determinations and insulin dose administration, Melanie's blood sugars were beginning to stabilize, even though a routine dose schedule had not yet been established. Additionally, she could not yet be trusted to eat properly. Candy bar wrappers were found in her room on several occasions during the first 3 days of hospitalization.

In individual psychotherapy, Melanie was able to acknowledge that she "used to be mad" about her diabetes because it interfered with her social life. She found school "boring" and indicated that she was able to stay home much of the time because "nobody hassled me to go." When confronted in group psychotherapy that she appeared to be feeling sorry for herself, she replied angrily, "You don't know what it's like to have this [expletive] disease!"

Treatment Team Evaluation

The treatment team adjusted the severity ratings of Melanie's impairments based on her behaviors and consensually agreed that the patient objectives defined for her at the beginning of her care were still reasonable and could be met by time of discharge. Behaviors identified in the clinical update demonstrated some progress in meeting her patient objectives. The bracketed percentages following each of the patient objectives in the treatment plan record the team's decision of Melanie's progress toward meeting each one of them.

The psychiatrist identified an endogenous component to her depression and recommended that she be given a trial on antidepressant medication. Melanie was started on fluoxetine, 20 mg once a day. Psychological testing revealed that Melanie was in fact a very thoughtful young woman with a capacity for introspection and insight into her difficulties. The interventions for individual psychotherapy were modified based on that information. The team also agreed that family therapy would be required for Melanie's impairments of Dysphoric Mood and Truancy to drop in severity. Despite her habitual Truancy, Melanie appeared capable of profiting from cognitive treatment interventions.

Patient Impairment Profile Patient: Melanie W.

Impairment	Severity Rating 2/9	2/12	Interim Goal
1. **Suicidal Thought/Behavior**	4	4	2
2. **Dysphoric Mood**	4	4	2
3. **Concomitant Medical Condition (juvenile-type diabetes mellitus)**	4	3	3
4. **Inadequate Healthcare Skills**	2	2	—
5. **Family Dysfunction**	2	2	—
6. **Truancy**	2	2	—

Progress Toward Patient Objectives

(To Be Met by Discharge: 3/2/95)

(* = Target Objective)

Suicidal Thought/Behavior

Patient will verbalize:

- Plans to harm oneself rather than act on them. **[25%]**
- The precipitants for Suicidal Thought/Behavior. **[25%]**
- Alternative actions to be taken when feeling suicidal. [0%]
- Reasons for living. [0%]

* Warning signs that Suicidal Thought/Behavior is exacerbating. [0%]

* A plan of action to be taken should Suicidal Thought/Behavior exacerbate. [0%]

Patient will demonstrate:

- Participation in a prescribed treatment program. **[50%]**
- Commitment to a behavioral contract not to harm oneself. **[25%]**

* Elimination of Suicidal Thought/Behavior. **[25%]**

* A completed self-care (discharge) plan, including steps to be taken should Suicidal Thought/Behavior return or exacerbate. [0%]

Dysphoric Mood

Patient will verbalize:

- Awareness of severe mood changes when they occur. [0%]
- Awareness of the precipitating factors for negative mood changes. [0%]
- Statements that are positive and hopeful rather than negative and self-deprecating. [0%]

* Warning signs that the Dysphoric Mood is exacerbating. [0%]
* A plan of action to be taken should the Dysphoric Mood exacerbate. [0%]

Patient will demonstrate:

- Participation in a prescribed treatment program. **[25%]**
- Increased self-initiated and self-directed activities. **[25%]**
- Increased integrating behaviors with others. **[25%]**

* Reduction in the Dysphoric Mood as evidenced by a 50% decrease in the Hamilton Rating Scale for Depression (rated at the initiation of treatment) and/or a 50% improvement in the Coopersmith Self-Esteem Inventory. [0%]
* A completed self-care (discharge) plan, including steps to be taken should the Dysphoric Mood return or exacerbate. [0%]

Concomitant Medical Condition (juvenile-type diabetes mellitus)

Patient will verbalize:

- Thoughts and feelings regarding the medical condition. **[25%]**

* Acceptance of responsibility for management of the medical condition. [0%]
* Warning signs that the medical condition is exacerbating. **[25%]**
* A plan of action to be taken should the medical condition exacerbate. **[25%]**

Patient will demonstrate:

- Adherence to the treatment regimen for the medical condition (e.g., self-initiated medication compliance, self-selected appropriate diet). [0%]

* A self-care worksheet that describes the medical condition, its etiology, prognosis, treatment regimen, and potential future complications. [0%]
* Adequate management of the medical condition. **[25%]**

Progress Toward Patient Objectives

(To Be Met by the End of Treatment: 7/10/95)

Inadequate Healthcare Skills

Patient will verbalize:

- Acceptance of responsibility for the Inadequate Healthcare Skills. [0%]
- Warning signs that the healthcare skills are deteriorating. [0%]
- A plan of action to be taken should healthcare skills deteriorate. [0%]

Patient will demonstrate:

- Adherence to the treatment program for the Inadequate Healthcare Skills. **[25%]**
- A self-care worksheet that describes the specific healthcare issues needing to be addressed. [0%]
- The ability to bathe, brush teeth, comb hair, and wear clean clothes daily. **[50%]**
- The ability to select nutritious foods from the four food groups at mealtime. **[25%]**
- Adequate healthcare skills. **[25%]**

Family Dysfunction

Patient will verbalize:

- Understanding of each family member's role in the Family Dysfunction. [0%]
- Awareness of the patient's own dysfunctional roles within the family. [0%]
- A plan for modifying the patient's own role within the family. [0%]
- The warning signs that the family is again becoming dysfunctional. [0%]
- A contingency plan of action to be taken should the Family Dysfunction increase. [0%]

Patient will demonstrate:

- Discussion with family members regarding each other's dysfunctional roles. [0%]
- A written clarification of the "nonnegotiables" for each family member. [0%]

- A written family contract that specifies the plans for change in the Family Dysfunction and the actions to be taken when significant disagreement occurs. [0%]
- Adherence to a written family contract. [0%]
- Elimination of distressing Family Dysfunction. [0%]

Truancy

Patient will verbalize:

- The precipitants for truant behaviors. **[25%]**
- Acceptance of responsibility for the Truancy. **[25%]**
- An alternative plan of action to take when thoughts to be truant occur. [0%]

Patient will demonstrate:

- A written paper that identifies the precipitating factors and the adverse consequences of being truant. [0%]
- Successful negotiation of a contract with the family regarding the consequences of continued Truancy. [0%]
- Meeting with an educator/counselor to develop a plan/contract for repairing the specific educational deficits resulting from Truancy. [0%]
- Adherence to the family contract regarding school/work attendance. [0%]
- Elimination of Truancy. [0%]

Case 2: Bob D.

Clinical Update

By the third hospital day, Bob was no longer experiencing any Delusions. After three 10-mg doses of haloperidol during his first 12 hours on the inpatient unit, Bob was calm, occasionally dozed off, and he reported to some staff and several peers that he had been "tripping out." A urine drug screen revealed the presence of phencyclidine (PCP), and he acknowledged that he had in fact taken "a hit of dust" an hour before the onset of his bizarre behavior prior to admission. The antipsychotic medication was subsequently discontinued. Bob detailed that he was in fact a frequent user of PCP (two to three times a week) and was drinking up to a case of beer a day. On several occasions since coming into the hospital, he stated that he felt unable to stop himself from abusing drugs and alcohol.

Although at times Bob felt anxious and restless on the unit, he showed no physical signs of alcohol withdrawal thus far. Clinical assessments also revealed a conspicuous lack of ordinary problem-solving skills (e.g., how to use a telephone book). Bob was aware that he was very successful in persuading his wife or parents to balance his checkbook, make appointments for him, negotiate with creditors, renew his automobile insurance, and so on. Bob was now feeling ashamed about being so inadequate in managing these activities of daily living, and he was mortified to discover that other people were aware of his inadequacies and his drug and alcohol abuse. In group psychotherapy, however, Bob also questioned whether it was accurate to be labeled as an alcoholic "because alcoholics are people who don't want to stop drinking."

Treatment Team Evaluation

The team's consensus was that Bob was a highly narcissistic young man who had been able to exploit others at the expense of acquiring his own independent living skills. His painful feelings of inadequacy and vulnerability to any perceived criticism were regulated with alcohol and hallucinogens. Bob expressed some relief at no longer needing to maintain this charade in life, and he agreed to proceed with whatever treatment recommendations we had for him. Bob's reactions, observations, and comments about himself and his behavior looked like Tantrums but now came to be understood as the manifestation of his negative and self-deprecating view of himself and his feelings of futility about ever being able to change. The identification of the Self-Esteem Deficiency contributed to a more accurate understanding of Bob's clinical presentation—and would no doubt impact the treatment of his Substance Abuse. The severity of the Self-Esteem Deficiency on its own was felt to be a 2—destabilizing.

The team agreed that Bob's Substance Abuse was no longer an imminent danger but could very likely become so if he were not closely supervised, and, therefore, the severity rating of the Substance Abuse was dropped to 3. (Because the Delusions were quickly resolved and not anticipated to require further intervention at this time, their severity rating is 0.) The team recommended that Bob continue his inpatient treatment on the chemical dependency unit, where he would be monitored with an alcohol detoxification protocol.

Patient Impairment Profile Patient: Bob D.

Impairment	Severity Rating		
	9/1	9/4	Interim Goal
1. Delusions	**4**	**0**	**N/A**
2. Substance Abuse (Alcohol, PCP)	**4**	**3**	**2**
3. Tantrums	**2**	*****	**—**
4. Self-Esteem Deficiency	**—**	**2**	**—**
5. Inadequate Self-Maintenance Skills	**—**	**2**	**—**

*See #5.

Progress Toward Patient Objectives

(To Be Met by Discharge: 9/22/95)

(* = Target Objective)

Delusions (Nonparanoid)

Patient will verbalize:

- Awareness of the presence of delusional thinking. **[100%]**
- Responsibility for the presence of the Delusions. **[100%]**
- The precipitants for the delusional thinking. **[100%]**

* A plan of action to be taken should the Delusions exacerbate. **[N/A]**

Patient will demonstrate:

- Adherence to the medical treatment of the Delusions. **[100%]**

* Absence of Delusions for 72 hours. **[100%]**

- Adequate management of the Delusions. **[100%]**

* A completed self-care (discharge) plan, including steps to be taken should the Delusions return or exacerbate. **[N/A]**

Substance Abuse

Patient will verbalize:

- Acceptance of personal responsibility for the Substance Abuse. **[25%]**

- The precipitants for past Substance Abuse. **[25%]**
- The potential hazards of substance substitution. [0%]
- The warning signs that the urge to abuse is returning. [0%]

* A contingency plan of action to be taken should the urge to abuse persist. [0%]

* A plan of action to be taken should a relapse occur. [0%]

Patient will demonstrate:

- Adherence to a medication/treatment program for the Substance Abuse. **[25%]**
- Completion of "Step One," which satisfactorily records the adverse impact of the Substance Abuse on the patient's and others' lives. [0%]
- A three- to five-page paper that addresses Substance Abuse as a disease, the problems of substance substitution, the relapse indicators, and relapse avoidance techniques. [0%]
- Obtaining a 12-step program sponsor. [0%]

* Abstinence from substances of abuse as evidenced by negative, random urine drug screenings. **[25%]**

* A written ongoing self-care (discharge) plan for the Substance Abuse, including steps to be taken should a relapse occur or the urge to abuse exacerbate. [0%]

Progress Toward Patient Objectives

(To Be Met by the End of Treatment: 12/11/95)

Self-Esteem Deficiency

Patient will verbalize:

- Feelings of inadequacy and self-doubt. [0%]
- Awareness of heightened sensitivity to criticism. [0%]
- Positive attributes, strengths, and talents. [0%]
- Warning signs that self-esteem has been injured. [0%]

Patient will demonstrate:

- Ability to listen to criticism without "reacting." [0%]
- Ability to make a change or an improvement in response to criticism. [0%]
- Ability to repair injured self-esteem. [0%]

- A written self-care (discharge) plan for the Self-Esteem Deficiency, including steps to be taken should the deficiency exacerbate. [0%]

Inadequate Self-Maintenance Skills

Patient will verbalize:

- Adverse consequences of Inadequate Self-Maintenance Skills. [0%]
- Willingness to acquire necessary self-maintenance skills. [0%]

Patient will demonstrate:

- Utilization of the appropriate resources to acquire necessary self-maintenance skills. [0%]
- Adequate self-maintenance skills. [0%]
- A written self-care (discharge) plan for Inadequate Self-Maintenance Skills, including steps to be taken should future deficiencies become manifest. [0%]

Conclusion

Documenting the progress and outcome of the treatment addresses two aspects of accountability: 1) the practitioner is competent, and 2) the treatment is effective. The decisions as to which treatment services are going to be provided will soon be (and in some cases already are) determined by patient care algorithms. Hopefully, these "practice guidelines" will be derived from reliable outcome data. In Chapter 10, we describe trends in the healthcare marketplace and in information management that are driving the evolution of care management mechanisms in mental health. We also recommend that practitioners locate their nearest access ramps to the healthcare information superhighway. Although we are not sure where it is going either, we are confident it will be the only way to get there.

Chapter 10

Managing the Future of Managed Care

"We will no longer be accepting paper claims."

In this chapter, we review the role of marketplace principles in shaping managed mental healthcare models. Consumers' expectation for quality healthcare services with good outcomes and purchasers' demand for healthcare value—quality at a reasonable cost—are addressed as the mental health practitioner's new challenge to meet. The application of automated information management systems for providing value and improving quality is endorsed, and implications of electronic network communication systems for mental healthcare delivery models are discussed.

Discussing the future of managed mental healthcare recalls an anecdote from history as a context for understanding the practitioners' experience with managed care review. When the king of France, Louis XVI, was told of a plot to seize control of the palace and overthrow the monarchy, he asked the Duke of Orleans, "Is this a revolt?" "No," the duke assured the king, "it's a revolution." When case management interrupted traditional indemnity reimbursement for mental health services, many practitioners felt as if they too were witness to a plot—a crafty insurance payers' tactic to seize a share of their fees and sentence them to a lifetime of paperwork and time-consuming tournaments of telephone tag. The fact is, however, that the emergence of managed care was neither a spontaneous gesture nor an isolated innovation devised by a few insurgent healthcare carriers.

Negotiating agreements with healthcare providers to reduce fees (in return for additional referrals as "preferred providers") was the private insurers' first effort to stem the skyrocketing cost of United States healthcare—or at least their stake in it. Early managed care mechanisms were nascent attempts at economic reform of healthcare delivery and, as such, the harbinger of an inevitable overhaul and restructuring of healthcare financing in this country. Although the time frame for such comprehensive reform is yet to be determined, "managed care" will navigate into the future on the same powerful undercurrents that will be steering the course of healthcare delivery reform.

Compelling facts underscore the urgency for change. As of December 1994, 41 million Americans lacked healthcare coverage, and the worrisome economic prediction is that by the year 2000 more than 20% of the population from ages 21–65 will be uninsured unless broad reform measures are undertaken (American Medical Association 1995). The more dire predicament in healthcare is its cost, which has spun out of control since World War II. In the 1950s, an average stay in an acute hospital required about 2 weeks of work for the median-income American family. In 1990, despite a lower likelihood of being hospitalized and a shorter length of stay, the same median income family had to work more than 7 weeks to pay for one acute admission (D. E. Grant 1994). In the 1950s, getting sick meant a loss of wages; in the 1990s, getting sick means possibly facing the leading cause of personal financial catastrophe—medically induced bankruptcy (Barlett and Steele 1992).

No longer shielded from the escalating expenditures for healthcare by traditional indemnity insurance, patients are becoming healthcare shoppers and, as such, make decisions about what to buy and what to pass over. Now that patients are concerned about the cost of healthcare, they will influence how and what care will be delivered. Interestingly, the choices that patients will make are knowable because their decisions are predetermined by predictable supply-and-demand principles of a marketplace. For participants in the future managed care, this is an important fact to recognize and keep in mind.

Mental Healthcare in a Competitive Consumer Marketplace

For any business enterprise, gloomy facts such as those discussed above signal what economists refer to as "market failure." The federal legislation and economic manipulations that will ultimately be prescribed to heal the ailing United States healthcare system remain unknown. What has been definitely established, however, is that healthcare is a business, a big business. It commands one-seventh of the nation's resources, provides one-eleventh of all jobs, and has central importance to all labor-management negotiations by being the most prized benefit for seven-eighths of all employed persons (D. E. Grant 1994). Although contrary to the centuries-old legacies of medical ethics, fiduciary responsibility, and social beneficence in medicine, healthcare has become a commercialized and competitive industry. It is no longer prudent for mental health practitioners to see themselves as being outside the competitive fray that characterizes the consumer marketplace. They need to understand the implications of "peddling their wares" in a venue teeming with quality-conscious consumers and value-conscious purchasers.[1]

Traditional fiduciary accountability of practitioners to their patients has been augmented to include their fiscal accountability as a sup-

[1] An engaging and detailed review of the economic evolution of healthcare in this country since the Civil War—as well as a fascinating account of the powerful interest groups and federal legislation that inadvertently produced this healthcare crisis—can be found in *Reforming the Health Care Marketplace* (Drake 1994).

plier/provider to a consumer/patient. Business education training modules in medical schools, graduate psychology programs, and residency training programs are becoming the norm as students are taught how to assess their professional identity and determine professional goals, make informed employment choices, and understand how their clinical and management decisions affect others in complex organizations. Several training programs have recently adopted a new physician's oath for graduating students of medicine. This oath includes "the duty to be the patient's advocate on matters related to insurance and other financial impediments which may interfere with receiving care" (L. Lasagna 1984 as quoted in Altman 1990, p. B6).

Any or all of the changes that have occurred (e.g., commercialization, "monetarization," privatization, the rise of the new medical industrial complex) may be contrary to the traditional conceptions of professionalism and patient-service orientation held by healthcare providers. Nevertheless, the significant result of these changes is that healthcare delivery is now oriented to performance and, as such, is subservient to the value-quality-cost ratio and basic economic principles of supply and demand. When a business (e.g., healthcare) has a surplus of supplies (e.g., practitioners and services) and the demand (patient use of services) is high, strategic how-to-win-business tactics based on performance data and supply-and-demand principles prevail. The stage is set for active competition in the healthcare marketplace.

What a competitive marketplace can mean for the winners is stunningly illustrated in mental health's own backyard. Just a few short years ago, a handful of external review companies began overseeing the utilization of inpatient mental health benefits. These review companies have since coalesced and mushroomed into major players in the healthcare marketplace and now make up a managed behavioral care industry that publishes its own *Annual Market Share Journal* and generates yearly revenues (in 1994) of more than $1.9 billion. Aggressive marketing and strategic competitive pricing explain why 45.9% of the estimated 222 million Americans with health insurance are now enrolled in some type of managed behavioral health program (Oss 1994).

Managed Care or Managed Delivery?

Managed care has been characterized as any outside influence on the practitioner-patient relationship that a practitioner does not like (Goodman

1994). For our purposes, a narrower definition of managed care is the overseeing of the process of care—that is, monitoring the nature, intensity, and duration of treatment interventions (and, in mental healthcare, which disciplines ought to provide them). Managed care also includes measuring compliance with accepted clinical standards and well-researched practice guidelines for predetermined conditions and their combinations. (A comprehensive treatment database to create practice guidelines for all mental health conditions, however, does not exist at this time.)

There are those who predict that managed care review as currently conducted in mental health will be obsolete within 5 years. The cost and time of telephone-conducted review has become too burdensome for all concerned, and a paper-based review through traditional communication channels wastes too many valuable days. Provider organizations are overwhelmed by the task of credentialing providers and biennially updating thousands of practitioner files. Who, then, will manage the future of managed care? Hopefully, the managed care companies themselves predict the answer in their treatment authorization letters to their providers. Invariably, they contain this (or some similar) disclaimer: "The ultimate decision regarding the treatment is of course the responsibility of the beneficiary and the treatment provider."

To manage means to have charge of, conduct, handle, or administer. Management of patient care has been and will continue to be the responsibility—a duty of care—of the provider. For some of the reasons described, managed care companies have become more interested in identifying low-risk, cost-effective key providers or provider groups who can be relied on to demonstrate good patient outcomes with minimal or no case management. Some managed care companies are seeking to define "anchor groups" of practitioners on whom they can depend to provide a broad range of services within specific geographic areas and be creative and innovative with newer treatment alternatives. These anchor groups will operate with a minimum amount of micromanagement.

Providers are being profiled by marketplace performance criteria (e.g., practitioner costs, availability, timeliness, recidivism, patient satisfaction). Providers who can convincingly provide better value for the healthcare dollar, by demonstrating improvement in both efficient performance and good patient outcomes, will maintain their competitive edge. The brisk sales of "point of service" health maintenance organization (HMO) plans—which offer an increase in out-of-pocket expense for the option to utilize out-of-network providers—confirm what consumer surveys have suggested: patients are concerned about the quality of their healthcare and are willing to pay extra for more personal attention to their needs and for perceived superior quality. It is unlikely that this consumer orientation will change significantly in the near future.

Mental health practitioners may be able to rescue some of their autonomy and decision making if they possess the business management and marketplace skills to do so. Successfully competing in a business inevitably requires power. Knowledge is power in a marketplace, and aggregated well-analyzed information significantly enhances a knowledge base. The data requirements necessary for offering optimal value, improving efficiency, and demonstrating good patient outcomes are demanding. Electronic data systems and communication networks will be required; similar technological capability soon also will be a requirement for participation in managed mental health networks.

The functional relationship between value and quality is that one enhances the other. Information management and network system skills enhance both of them. Quality, value, and information management are essential skills for successfully competing in the sophisticated healthcare marketplace. Effectively managing the future of managed care necessitates that attention be paid to these three areas, which are addressed individually in the next sections.

Managing the Management of Care

Value Management

Webster's *New World Dictionary* defines *value* as "the worth of a thing in money or goods at a certain time" or "that which is thought of as more or less desirable, useful, estimable, important." Supply-and-demand economics in the marketplace defines value as the quotient of the quality of a product divided by the cost of a product:

$$\text{Value} = \frac{\text{Quality}}{\text{Cost}}$$

Responding to the purchasers' demand for value, therefore, can be accomplished—using this equation—by improving quality or reducing cost.

Patient outcome as a measure for demonstrating quality is the new focus for many managed care organizations and insurance companies. Although favorable outcomes are a reasonable priority for purchasers and consumers, practitioners can proactively ensure that clinical outcome is not promulgated as the *only* measure of quality and therefore value. An aspect of quality referred to as *perceptive quality* can enhance value as well (perceptive quality is one of three aspects of quality described in the next section). Perceptive quality is "that degree of excellence which is perceived by the recipient or the observer of care rather than by the provider of care" (J. Brown 1995, p. 5). Practitioners can facilitate the perception of quality by the reviewer through clear documentation and accurate, timely articulation of the process of treatment. Patients perceive value in services that respond and adapt to their individualized needs and preferences. In a service business marketplace, the most important gauge for what needs to be provided, how well it is being provided, and whether it can be done better is the consumers' perception of the providers' services.

Providing value becomes leverage in a competitive market. In the typical growth and maturity phases of an industry marketplace, either costs must decline or product value must increase. Two examples of mental health delivery models that aim to provide a better dollar value by reducing overall cost of care are 1) integrated delivery systems and 2) independent practice associations (IPAs).

Integrated delivery is a newer competition feature for some HMOs and large managed care organizations that are turning away from benefit "carve-out" companies (traditional specialty managed care companies) to newer "carve-in" companies for providing mental health and substance abuse treatment. Carve-out companies manage a predetermined amount of behavioral health benefits in return for a fee that may or may not include third-party administrator functions (paying the providers). Carve-in companies are intended to work more closely with primary healthcare providers and usually manage mental healthcare within the same healthcare benefit package of its parent company (Parker 1995).

One well-known managed mental healthcare company requires its providers to make telephone contact with the patient's primary care physician, request and review the patient's medical records, and, in return, provide the primary care physician with a written report of the initial assessment, regular progress summaries, notice of any changes in the treatment plan, and a discharge summary. While these additional responsibilities might feel like an unnecessary burden, the trend in managed behavioral care appears to be this: true integration between behavioral healthcare and physical healthcare is essential in order to provide quality and efficient care.

Vertically integrated delivery is the sequential linking of provider services and settings at all stages of the treatment—from brief and infrequent medication management visits to intensive inpatient services. This model is agreeably more cost efficient, provides better quality care by maintaining continuity, and, hence, is a better value. Anchor groups (referred to previously) become even more desirable when they can be relied on to provide a broad scope of services.

While HMOs and managed care organizations are now energetically competing for larger contracts covering more millions of lives, a number of practitioner groups are now entering the competition with the belief that their own networks can provide even better value for the mental healthcare dollar. The most appealing networks consist of provider groups large enough to provide a broad range of integrated treatment services. These groups refer to themselves as IPAs. IPAs are self-regulated incorporated group practices composed (for our purposes) of various mental health professionals. They seek contracts with managed care organizations (e.g., HMOs, insurers, self-insured employers). IPAs agree to accept a predetermined fee for providing treatment services for a large group of members regardless of how much medical care that group needs. This flat per member–per month fee is known in the insurance industry as *capitation.*

These are the first provider-created models that have the capability to compete with the HMOs, which had the head start in the managed care marketplace. To track and provide both cost-efficient and quality care without incurring additional (expensive) risks, IPAs devise their own innovative mechanisms for approving, providing, and concurrently managing all treatment services. Practitioners become "incentivized" to experiment with and identify the most cost-efficient alternative treatment strategies to achieve a given result. In the fully risk-shared capitation environment, where all providers share the same finance pool, such flexing of benefits, as well as active care coordination, is generally encouraged.

A very rich opportunity is now at hand to assess the quality and value of innovative and creative treatment approaches for specific clinical presentations. The need for reliable and serviceable treatment data to measure them systematically is obvious. We believe that the patient impairment profile (PIP)—impairments and their severity ratings—and patient objectives, accompanied by specific practitioner interventions (yet to be clearly defined), offer one of the best clinical databases for the ongoing measurement, assessment, and improvement of the quality, and ultimately the value, of mental healthcare.

Quality Management

The management of quality is first and foremost the responsibility of the practitioner. The practitioner identifies and interprets the patient's needs and recommends specific treatment. Practitioners are now, and will increasingly be, profiled on the basis of "quality data," including the traditional adverse occurrence indicators related to recidivism, complications, readmissions, and over- and underutilization data, as well as the newer "outcome data." But quality management is also the responsibility of the *team* in managed care, which includes, at a minimum, the practitioner, other providers of care, the reviewer and/or the coordinator of care, and the payer.

Quality is notoriously difficult to define as a stand-alone concept. Quality is the degree of excellence of a product or service and therefore can exist only in a context of comparison. Consider the following example: A 22-year-old single male who was physically abused as a child before being diagnosed with dyslexia seeks therapy because "I'm totally useless—what kind of future could I ever have?" Should he see a social worker, a psychologist, or a psychiatrist? Whom should he choose to ensure that he receives quality care? Each discipline might reasonably claim to have expertise in one or more of the potential problem areas for this patient. Who is better skilled at assessing and treating adult dyslexia? Who is better skilled at working with adult victims of child abuse? Who is the most skillful at assessing the potential for suicide in overtly depressed individuals? Without naming the specific attributes for comparing the three practitioners, the question of whom to see for the "best-quality care" is unanswerable. Many healthcare speakers (and politicians) take advantage of this relational feature of quality when they quip, "I can't define quality either, but I know it when I see it."

Although difficult to grab, embrace, and understand as an abstraction, quality in healthcare begins to get more concrete when one looks at its three aspects: measurable, appreciative, and perceptive (J. Brown 1995). *Measurable quality* is generally defined as compliance with, or adherence to, standards. We assume that quality can be adequately, if not completely, measured once practitioners define the standards of care under which they can comfortably practice.

Appreciative quality is the comprehension and appraisal of excellence beyond minimal standards and criteria, requiring the sometimes even nonarticulate judgments of skilled, experienced practitioners and sensitive, caring persons. Peer review bodies rely on the judgments of like professionals in determining the quality or nonquality of specific patient-practitioner interactions. Courts of law use expert witnesses to determine whether professional behavior was "reasonable" or "negligent," words of judgment that reach beyond the purely measurable.

Perceptive quality is the degree of excellence that is perceived by the recipient or the observer of care rather than by the provider of care ("I know it when I see it—or feel it."). To manage quality well within these three aspects, practitioners must measure themselves or be measured against approved standards, must utilize peers and comparative data to assess and improve, and must deal effectively and positively with patients and other observers to promote their satisfaction with care and services.

The Joint Commission on Accreditation of Healthcare Organizations, in its own pursuit of quality and clear definition, first revised the 1994 hospital standards and then all other accreditation program standards to incorporate both utilization and risk issues under the umbrella of quality or what is now called "performance improvement." The accrediting body looks at nine different attributes of quality as "dimensions of performance":

> Performance is *what* is done and *how well* it is done to provide health care. The level of performance in health care is the degree to which *what* is done is *efficacious* and *appropriate* for the individual patient; and the degree to which it is *available* in a *timely* manner to patients who need it; *effective, continuous* with other care and care providers; *safe, efficient,* and *caring* and *respectful* of the patient. (Joint Commission on Accreditation of Healthcare Organizations 1995, p. 241, emphases in original)

It *is* possible to manage these dimensions of quality or performance. We can develop measures of performance for each of these dimensions as they are relevant to improvement of our mental healthcare systems or processes. We can measure (collect, aggregate, and display) data to learn what is better or even best practice; what can be improved when compared with other systems, processes, or practices; and what needs more in-depth assessment. Through appropriate comparative, and perhaps intensive, assessment of the data, we gain understanding of current practice patterns. Only then do we have good, accurate information to use in making viable improvement decisions.

Quality management is about comparative measurement, the judgments of peers, and the perceptions of recipients and observers of care.

It is all-encompassing and requires us to measure, assess, and improve over time all the dimensions of performance, our utilization of resources, and the degree of patient and organizational risk. According to Avedis Donabedian (1980, 1982), an epidemiologist, quality management is also about structure, process, and outcome.

Donabedian (1980, 1982) referred to structure, process, and outcome as the kinds of information we use to draw inferences about the quality of care, merely because they are causally related: structure leads to process leads to outcome. Today's buzzword, *outcome,* is touted—and perhaps rightfully so—as a key indicator of value in healthcare. It is dependent on, and results from, effective process and structure. In managed care, structure may refer to the benefit plan, contract arrangements, policies, staffing arrangements, staff and practitioner qualifications, and so on. Process includes all procedures (e.g., referral, routine access, after-hours or emergency access, authorization, provision of care, communication, billing) as well as the many steps that make up each process. Outcome refers to the results of actual care rendered or the effects of support processes.

Even when the causal relationships between structure, process, and outcome are fully understood, as indicators of quality they are more probabilities than certainties, due to the ever-present individual variables called patients and practitioners. Donabedian (1980, 1982) stratified possible outcomes of healthcare into

- Clinical (symptoms, diagnosis, disease staging, diagnostic performance)
- Physical/physiological (abnormalities, functional performance)
- Psychological/psychosocial (feelings, beliefs, knowledge, impairments, behaviors, role performance)
- Integrative (mortality, longevity with or without impairments, monetary value/costs)
- Evaluative (customer opinions, satisfactions, dissatisfactions)

The term *outcomes management* was actually coined by Paul Ellwood, founder of InterStudy, located in Excelsior, Minnesota. He presented the concept as part of the "Shattuck Lecture: Outcomes Management: A Technology of Patient Experience," which was reprinted in the *New England Journal of Medicine* (Ellwood 1988). Ellwood used the term to refer to a "technology of patient experience designed to help patients, payers, and providers make rational medical [or mental health] care-related choices based on better insight into the effect of these choices on the patient's life" (p. 1551). To Ellwood, "the centerpiece and unifying ingredient" (p. 1552) of outcomes management is the tracking and measurement of the patient's functionality and well-being or quality of life.

Effective outcomes management will consist of

- A common language of mental health outcomes, understood by practitioners and patients
- A national database containing data and analysis on clinical, financial, and mental health outcomes and providing probability information about relationships between practitioner interventions and outcomes, as well as between outcomes and money spent
- An opportunity for decision makers to access analysis information relevant to choices that must be made

Ellwood believes that outcomes management is dependent on other developing techniques:

- Practitioner commitment to, and reliance on, standards and guidelines in selecting appropriate interventions
- Routine and systematic measurement of the functioning and well-being of patients, along with specific clinical outcomes, at appropriate time intervals
- Pooling of clinical and outcome data on a massive scale for comparison
- Analysis and dissemination of results from whatever segment of the database is pertinent to the decision maker

Our goal is that the data available through the PIP, patient objectives, and practitioner interventions will provide practitioners, practitioner groups, and mental healthcare organizations, including managed care organizations, with a rich clinical database for measurement, assessment, and improvement of the quality of mental healthcare at all levels. The clinical data set represented by this documentation method, when aggregated and appropriately analyzed over time as a large comparative database, should provide enough objective information to

- Establish a common language of mental health outcomes by linking patient progress in meeting impairment-specific objectives with actual reductions in severity ratings

- Formulate "practice guidelines" based not on practitioner or managed care organization opinion, but on actual clinical results or outcomes
- Develop and track the effectiveness of clinical pathways
- Make appropriate choices about level of care and intensity and type of treatment for particular PIPs
- Identify better and best practices based on relationships between patient progress in meeting objectives, reductions in severity ratings, practitioner interventions, and associated costs
- Select appropriate practitioners for particular PIPs based on effective interventions rather than educational background or reimbursement rates alone

Practitioners, groups, facilities, and all types of managed care organizations should benefit from participation in such a reference database. Certainly, access to clinical outcome data and information for decision making is a solid value. We also believe that, with some additional effort on the part of caregivers and support staff, other automated patient data will provide extremely valuable information concerning the efficiency, timeliness, and effectiveness of various managed care and direct care processes. We must have the ongoing, on-line capability to track and trend process issues such as referral and first visits, missed appointments, emergency calls, against-medical-advice discharges, readmissions, complaints, complications, medication side effects/adverse drug reactions, concomitant medical conditions, various combinations of impairments and severities, various combinations of impairments and practitioner interventions, best practices, and so on. Obviously, we are supporting the development of a fully automated clinical record. We believe that the future of mental healthcare lies in the management of both quality and value and in the management of information based on objective, accurate, well-defined, fully integrated clinical and nonclinical data.

Information Management

The data requirements necessary to compete effectively in today's healthcare marketplace far exceed the information that can usually be extracted from paper-based clinical records (and probably exceed what clinicians can reasonably be expected to provide in a handwritten record as well). If one longitudinal clinical record—which included the patient's entire medical history, psychological history, PIP, all laboratory studies, medication history, and charge data—were available for viewing at any time of the day or night, at home or in the office, the paper clinical record would theoretically become obsolete. If collections of uniformly documented clinical records were aggregated electronically for an analysis of the relationship between one or two clinical variables and patient outcomes, calling the medical records department to locate a particular group of records would be like telephoning a friend using two paper cups and a piece of string in a world of cellular phones.

Systems for electronically accessing a longitudinal healthcare record that captures a patient's entire health history from birth until death have been in various planning phases for over a decade. The Medical Records Institute was formed in 1981 to create national standards for electronic patient record systems and to be a bridge between the efforts of the United States and Europe. "Patient cards," which are credit-card–size health identification cards that contain a summary of a patient's entire medical history with present and previous medications and most recent laboratory studies, including X rays and electrocardiogram tracings, have been in use in some European countries for almost that long. A recent *Psychiatric Times* headline read "Psychiatry Needs Technology Now," and the article went on to report that it

> will be incumbent upon most behavioral care practitioners to technologize their offices and become computer literate. Insurance companies and managed care companies are moving toward requiring communication through a variety of technological modalities other than telephone or mail. They are working toward a system that will eventually use only electronic transmission of information. (Weil and Rosen 1994, p. 37)

Although there is not an exact timetable for this new system, experts suggest it is happening now.

Precedent for determining a national standard for electronic billing has already been set. Medicare carriers announced in early 1995 that of the more than 450 proprietary electronic claim-filing formats available nationwide, they will be accepting only two of them for processing electronic media claims filed by providers. (The two formats selected by Medicare are the National Standard Format and the American National Standards Institute. Additional information about these formats is available from Medicare.) Private insurers are anticipated to follow this lead.

In 1993, Medicare informed California-based contracted providers that billings submitted nonelectronically would be subject to up to a 24-day delay in processing. As of June 1996, Medicare in California no longer accepts paper claims but assists providers who are ready to convert to electronic billing.

How can automated clinical records impact the managed care review process? Imagine the following scenario for the second case example, Bob D., presented in the previous chapters: A facsimile transmittal or voice mail message is delivered by a managed care organization requesting a mental health provider (MHP) to assess a new patient. The managed care organization has also transmitted a preliminary PIP produced by a case manager using PIP-based software. The MHP sends back an electronic mail "yes" and within 10 minutes receives a complete patient identification block of information opening the clinical record as well as the ledger, billing forms, laboratory and referral request forms, and so on. This is accompanied by an initial treatment authorization.

After assessing the patient, the MHP returns to the screen, scrolls the impairment dictionary, and uses a mouse to "click" on the patient's impairments evidenced in the initial evaluation. The practitioner then clicks on the impairments that will be the focus of treatment (Figure 10–1).

A help screen is then displayed, which lists the qualifiers for all severity ratings for each identified impairment. The MHP clicks on the appropriate severity rating and enters a patient behavior to corroborate that rating (Figure 10–2).

A well-documented PIP is now complete (Figure 10–3).

The treatment goals are recorded next—simply by clicking on the anticipated reduction in severity for each impairment in the patient's profile by the time of discharge from that particular treatment setting. The practitioner enters the anticipated target date for this reduction in severity (Figure 10–4).

Next, the screen displays a list of patient objectives for each impairment, and the MHP selects those to be included in the treatment plan (or creates others) (Figure 10–5).

Next, a dictionary of interventions for each impairment is displayed, and the MHP again selects those to be implemented first (or adds others). The system automatically batches any impairments, severity qualifiers, or patient objectives newly created by the practitioner for later possible inclusion in the software's fixed database.

The MHP transmits the completed patient treatment plan back to the managed care organization. (As discussed in Chapter 9, this docu-

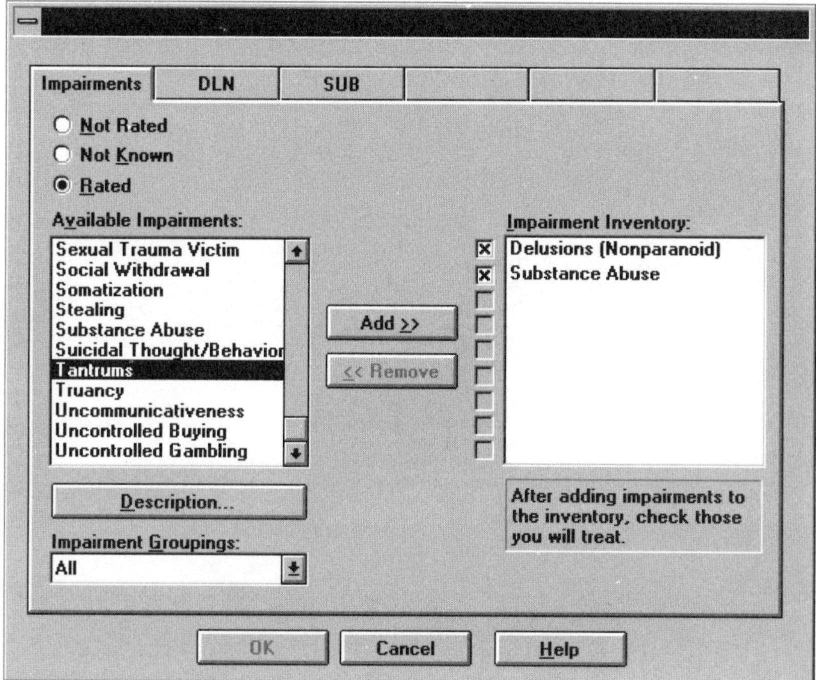

Community Sector Systems, Inc. PsychAccess™

Figure 10–1. Selecting the impairment.
Source. Copyrighted 1995 Community Sector Systems, Inc.

ment also expedites and simplifies the updating of the treatment plan as needed.) A confirmation of receipt of the plan is returned along with a treatment authorization. At the end of the month, in less time than it takes to pull a ledger card, type a bill, prepare an envelope, and stamp and mail it, an electronic claim is submitted with the click of the mouse, and notification of direct deposit to the MHP's bank is received back within hours.

Computerization of the clinical patient record is the "missing link" in an otherwise broad range of electronic data interchange systems available for healthcare. Although the national standard for computerized medical records has been in development for more than a decade, the mental healthcare profession has been given very little specific attention—largely because of the idiosyncratic documentation used in its clinical records. Unlike the rest of medicine, the stylized, personalized, and narrative text of mental health treatment documentation does not easily

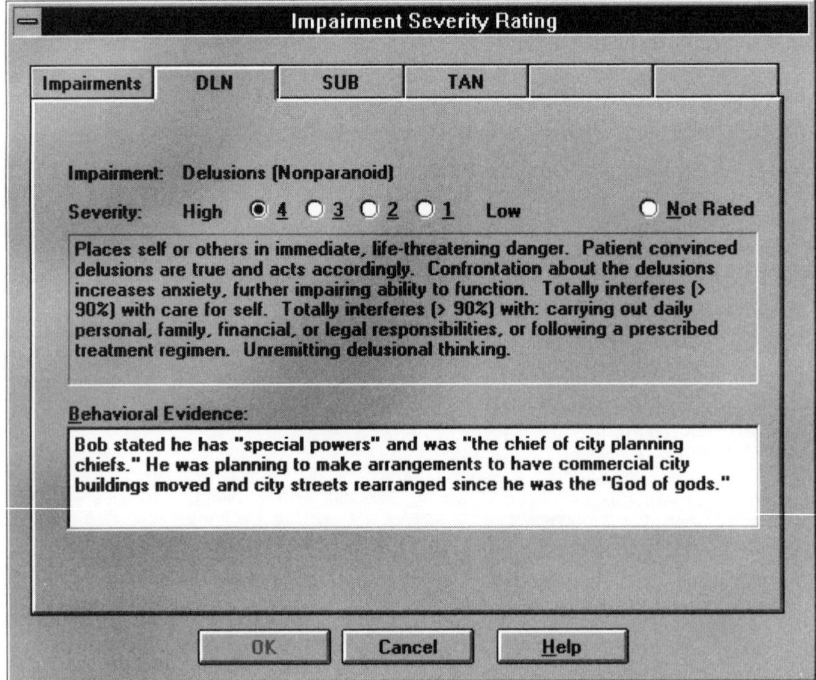

Figure 10–2. Rating the impairment severity.
Source. Copyrighted 1995 Community Sector Systems, Inc.

translate into discrete elements for the development of data sets. This was the impetus for us to create and develop the PIP-based method presented in this book.

Community Sector Systems (CSS), a communications software and systems integration development team located in Seattle, Washington, has produced state-of-the-art software capable of performing all the steps necessary to provide a complete treatment plan as well as a clinical treatment record that contains all the data that reviewers customarily require to authorize additional treatment services. This software—PsychAccess Clinical Information System—is available through CSS (1-800-988-6392). The data set structures discussed in this book—impairments, severity ratings, treatment goals, patient objectives, and practitioner interventions—are supported by the software. This software architecture is capable of revealing and analyzing interrelationships between clinical process elements such as demographic data, impairments, diagnosis, severity, pa-

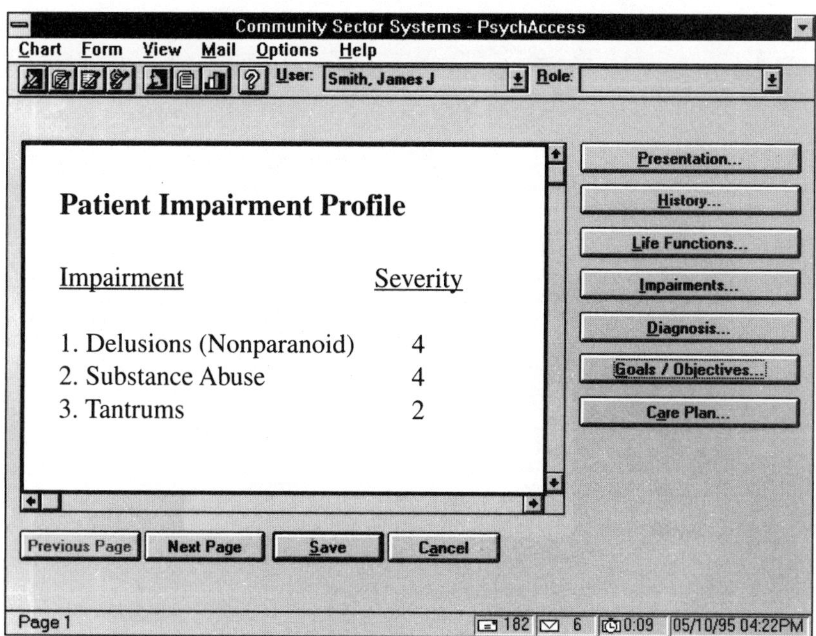

Figure 10–3. The patient impairment profile.
Source. Copyrighted 1995 Community Sector Systems, Inc.

tient objectives, treatment goals, interventions, medications, reasons for discharge, adverse occurrences, time frames, and charge data. This automated clinical record module was designed to link to accounting, benefit plan and contract information, outcomes analysis, patient scheduling, and care coordination modules that also will be available if the user does not have them in place already. When these provider systems are connected to clinics, hospitals, administrators, managed care companies, and payers, a fully integrated information system network for mental healthcare is established.

Healthcare professionals have been among the most technophobic white-collar business entities in this country. The newer information demands—which translate into time demands—are remedying this phobia by their sheer presence and magnitude. In *Living at Light Speed,* author Danny Goodman (1994) reminds us that the information superhighway not only will bring more changes into our lives on a daily basis, but it also will bring them to us more rapidly: "The better prepared we are for change, the less terrifying those changes are going to be" (p. 217). The technology is now here and waiting.

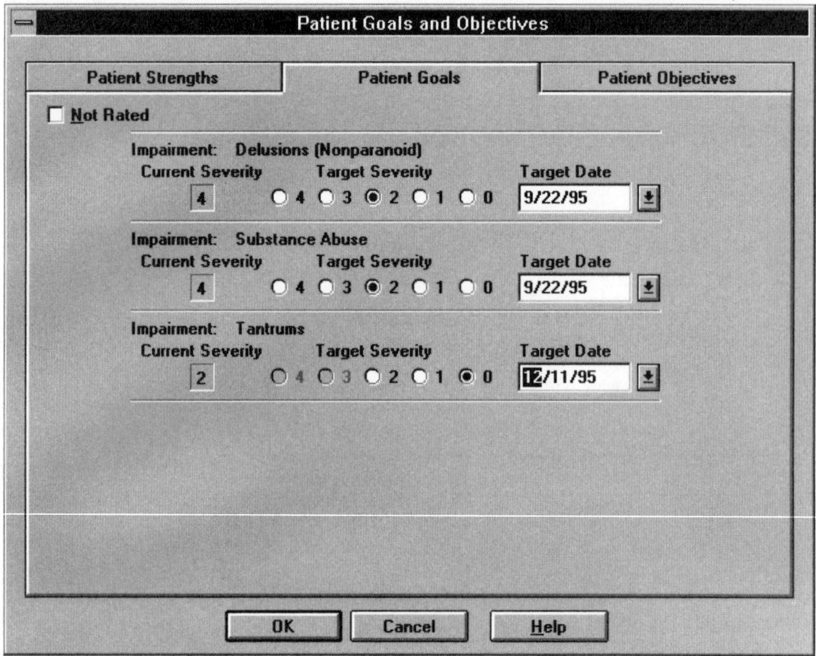

Figure 10–4. Determining treatment goals.
Source. Copyrighted 1995 Community Sector Systems, Inc.

Conclusion

The promise of automated information systems is exciting to contemplate. We believe that the skepticism and suspicions about software applications in a managed care environment are rooted in the concern about a basic premise of managed care review—namely, that treatment is objective enough for a person who has never seen or talked to the patient to rely on information about the patient to determine what services are appropriate. The underlying apprehension is that perhaps the most critical component of healthcare could slip away—or become managed away—in the (not ignoble) service of saving money. We are referring, of course, to that somewhat elusive and amorphous quality variously called compassion, humanitarianism, or caring. Recognizing individual differences in patients' needs, exercising discretion in a human interaction, and providing reassurance are essential "human" ingredients in healthcare delivery generally. These values are particularly pertinent for mental

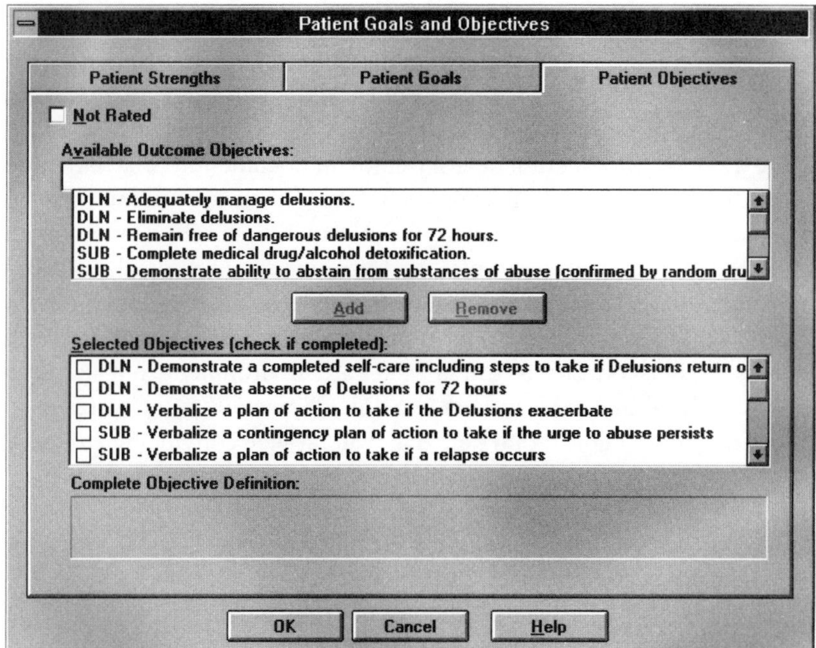

Figure 10–5. Selecting patient objectives.
Source. Copyrighted 1995 Community Sector Systems, Inc.

healthcare, and our commitment to technologizing treatment documentation is never intended to eclipse this fundamental bias. Yet, human qualities such as caring are not easy to describe, let alone reliably measure, validate, and analyze with a computer. Because they are so difficult to "see," both mental health and substance abuse treatment always seem to be under managed care's microscope. (This detailed overseeing of mental healthcare services on a day-by-day basis is what was referred to earlier as the micromanagement of care).

Mental health professionals "know" what quality mental healthcare is (the appreciative quality aspect of healthcare described earlier), and they also know when a patient has experienced a meaningful growth-enhancing treatment experience (articulated by the patient as the perceptive quality of care). Providing convincing evidence (measurable quality) to justify mental healthcare as a "real" and necessary component of a comprehensive human healthcare plan—to give it parity with the other medical specialties—requires a valid and reliable treatment language.

We propose that the PIP documentation method described in this book be considered as the basis for a national treatment documentation standard for mental health and substance abuse clinical records. One or more influential nationally based organizations need to establish and promote a standard for mental health treatment documentation to expedite aggregation of a clinical information database. This is a requirement for substantiating the known but as yet not quantitatively demonstrated clinical necessity, appropriateness, and effectiveness of mental health and substance abuse services for those who require them. As has been mentioned several times in this book, trust, reassurance, compassion, and caring are not contrary to a managed care environment, nor are they necessarily obliterated by automation. However, only systematic computer-ready clinical outcome data will provide convincing evidence that the "care" in healthcare—which is so much of what we hope mental healthcare is about—is a most essential and vital component of quality healthcare in general. This task can be a precedent-setting endeavor for the mental health profession.

That a computer decides whether to provide what a computer itself cannot provide—that is, human care—is an intriguing paradox of artificial intelligence technology. Fortunately, this does not intimidate a profession that often does its best work within a context of apparent contradiction. Mental healthcare practitioners, after all, endorse the challenge of a paradox every day—by permitting their patients to think the unthinkable, providing them safety to speak the unspeakable, and admiring their courage for managing the unmanageable.

Glossary

Acuity A description of the labor intensity component of care.

Appropriateness The degree to which the care provided is relevant to the patient's clinical needs, given the current state of knowledge; also, when the benefits of treatment outweigh the risks.

Assessment The systematic collection and analysis of the individual-specific data necessary to determine patient care needs, including at least the history, physical and mental status examinations, and any diagnostic tests or studies.

Clinical necessity Verification of the clinical need for appropriate treatment in the appropriate setting as evidenced by the patient's behaviors (statements and actions) and severity ratings.

Clinical rationale The relevance of the patient's behaviors to the identified impairments, or the stated behaviors and severity ratings to justify the identified impairments.

Critical impairment One of a predetermined subgroup of patient impairments that have the potential to justify more service-intensive treatment or settings (e.g., hospitalization).

Critical path A prospective, strategic treatment regimen or daily/intermittent regimen for patient care for a specified time period. A critical path identifies and integrates key functions and appropriate services to be provided by a multidisciplinary team for certain patient conditions.

Diagnosis A decision regarding the nature of a mental disorder (using DSM-IV or ICD-9-CM nomenclature) based on an examination of symptoms.

Discharge plan A prescribed course of action to be implemented when the patient is released or dismissed from a treatment setting or treatment, based on assessment of the patient's status and need for continuing care.

Goal *See* Treatment goal.

Impairment A behavior-based descriptor of patient dysfunction.

Impairment inventory The complete listing of identified impairments (*see* Patient impairment profile).

Indicator An objective measure of performance over time.

Information management Obtaining, analyzing, and using interpreted data to enhance and improve individual and organizational performance in patient care, governance, management, and support processes.

Intensity of service Total cost for a period of treatment, including personnel cost/hour, the personnel/patient ratio, the number of personnel hours, operational costs for the setting, and ancillary costs.

Intervention An action taken by a trained mental health professional to modify, resolve, or stabilize the patient's impairments.

Level of care The treatment setting (*see* Setting).

Objective *See* Patient objective.

Outcome The result of the performance or nonperformance of a process or processes of care.

Outcome measure An indicator (performance measure) that captures and quantifies the results of care.

Outcomes management The tracking and measurement of the patient's functionality and well-being resulting from choices made in rendering care to make improvements in future care choices and decisions.

Patient impairment profile (PIP) The impairments that are prioritized as the focus of treatment and their respective severity ratings.

Patient objective An anticipated patient statement or behavior that demonstrates progress toward repair of an impairment.

Patient outcome The individual-specific result of the performance or nonperformance of a process or process of care; the unique effect of care on the patient's functionality and well-being.

Performance measure A standard or indicator that captures and quantifies the performance of processes of care and their results or outcomes.

Practice guidelines Generally accepted principles for patient management, with care specifications based on the most current scientific findings (evidence of effectiveness), clinical expertise, and community standards of practice.

Practice parameters Overall patient management strategies that outline a range of appropriate services for a given clinical condition or identify a range of clinical conditions for which a given service may be appropriate, incorporating acceptable practice guidelines, clinical criteria, protocols, or standards of care.

Process of care A goal-directed, interrelated series of steps, actions, or mechanisms in the rendering of care.

Quality management A planned, systematic organization-wide approach to measure, assess, and improve performance, thereby continually improving the quality of patient care and services provided.

Setting A type of unit, facility, or other location where a treatment approach or modality is offered.

Severity of illness The degree of immediate risk of death or permanent loss of function due to an illness (general).

Severity rating A description of the degree of 1) danger or risk to self or others or 2) compromised function due to an impairment (for mental health impairments) (*see* Severity of illness).

Standard of care An indication of what "should" be done for a patient with a certain condition or problem (or the "usual" recommended care as defined by the American Hospital Association).

Target objective An anticipated patient statement or behavior that signals "discharge" to less service-intensive treatment.

Treatment goal The repair of an impairment or reduction in severity of an impairment to an endpoint or maintenance level. The anticipated reduction in impairment severity may be an *interim goal* or a *maintenance goal.*

Treatment modality A group or sequence of practitioner interventions employed as part of a therapeutic clinical service.

Treatment plan A patient clinical record that contains the assessment, diagnosis, patient impairment profile (including initial and updated severity ratings), patient objectives (with patient progress updates), treatment goals, interventions (initial and current), and discharge plan.

Value Perceived worth; the quotient of quality divided by the cost.

Value management The enhancement of perceived worth through a measurable improvement of quality or a decrease in cost (without a measurable reduction in quality) of a product or service.

Vertical integration The linking of treatment settings or services at all immediately related stages of (mental health) treatment.

Appendix A

Impairment Lexicon

* *Note to the reader: The impairments marked with an asterisk (*) are "critical impairments"—impairments that potentially can require more service-intensive treatment or an acute care setting.*

Alexithymia Impaired ability to label affect states (e.g., pleasure versus pain), differentiate them into more subtle shades of meaning, and communicate them to others.

Altered Sleep Any disruption of the normal 24-hour sleep-wake cycle, including insomnia, hypersomnia, early morning awakening, or night terrors.

***Anxiety** A state of uneasiness, worry, apprehension, or dread without sufficient objective justification (as distinguished from Obsessions, Pathological Guilt, and Phobia).

***Assaultiveness** Committing acts of physical violence that harm or potentially harm persons, property, or animals (as distinguished from Physical Abuse Perpetrator, Homicidal Thought/Behavior, and Sexual Trauma Perpetrator).

***Compulsions** Repetitive, stereotyped motor actions the individual does not want to perform and does not feel any pleasure in performing (as distinguished from Eating Disorders, Lying, Promiscuity, Sexual Object Choice Dysfunction, Substance Abuse, Uncontrolled Buying, and Uncontrolled Gambling). Failure to perform these actions results in increased Anxiety.

***Concomitant Medical Condition** Any pathophysiological disorder that requires or may require medical-surgical care (as distinguished from Medical Risk Factor).

Decreased Concentration Any observed or reported reduction in ability to direct one's thoughts or efforts to sustain attention.

***Delusions (Nonparanoid)** Beliefs obviously contrary to demonstrable fact.

***Delusions (Paranoid)** Systematic misbeliefs of persecution and grandeur obviously contrary to demonstrable fact.

***Dissociative States** Disturbances or alterations in the normally integrative functions of identity, memory, or consciousness (e.g., multiple personality, psychogenic amnesia or fugue, and depersonalization).

***Dysphoric Mood** Conscious and apparent psychic suffering characterized by sadness, gloominess, despair, or despondency.

***Eating Disorder** Gross disturbances in eating behavior, including binge eating, purging, abnormal weight gain or weight loss, and eating nonnutritive substances.

Educational Performance Deficit Academic deficiency not due to truancy or learning disability (e.g., functional illiteracy).

Egocentricity Excessive evaluation of things in terms of oneself and one's personal interests (e.g., excessive self-importance, arrogance, and empathic failures with others).

Emotional Abuse Perpetrator The perpetrator of deliberate nonphysical acts, including verbal abuse and emotional neglect, that are psychologically damaging to others.

Emotional Abuse Victim The victim of deliberate nonphysical acts, including verbal abuse and emotional neglect, that are psychologically damaging.

Encopresis Involuntary defecation after the age when sphincter control should have been attained (not due to a Concomitant Medical Condition).

Enuresis Involuntary passage of urine after the age when bladder control should have been attained (not due to a Concomitant Medical Condition).

Externalization and Blame Constant or inappropriate attributing of an intrapsychic function to an interpersonal experience (e.g., "I did what I did because 'he,' 'she,' or 'they' . . . ").

Family Dysfunction Insufficient knowledge of and failure to enact the expected and appropriate rights, responsibilities, and behaviors of parents and children; includes family role reversals and inadequate parents.

***Fire Setting** Persistent urges to set destructive fires.

Gender Dysphoria Confusion or discomfort with gender identity or role.

***Hallucinations** Sensory perceptions for which there are no external stimuli.

*Homicidal Thought/Behavior** Thoughts of or attempts at killing another human being.

***Inadequate Healthcare Skills** Deficient ability to take care of one's hygiene and basic personal health.

Inadequate Self-Maintenance Skills Inability to obtain and use relevant survival information in problem solving that compromises or endangers the quality of one's life; includes individuals who have inadequate social skills, make poor peer choices, or are pathologically dependent on others.

Learning Disability Achievement in arithmetic, writing, reading, expressive or receptive language, or speech that is markedly below expected level given the individual's schooling and intellectual capacity (measured by a standardized achievement test).

Lying Deliberate or uncontrolled falsification.

***Manic Thought/Behavior** Euphoric or intensely irritable mood, often with a grandiose quality, with restlessness, agitation, and increased number and speed of ideas (as distinguished from Mood Lability).

Manipulativeness Controlling or exploiting others solely to gain one's own ends.

Marital/Relationship Dysfunction Impaired marital or relationship functioning (due to either or both partners).

Marital/Relationship Dysfunction With Substance Abuse Impaired marital or relationship functioning (due to either or both partners) with a substance abuser.

***Medical Risk Factor** Any adverse reaction or other medical complication that could result from the initiation of a particular psychopharmacological intervention or electroconvulsive therapy (as distinguished from Concomitant Medical Condition).

Medical Treatment Noncompliance Failure to follow medical treatment recommendations.

***Mood Lability** Fluctuations in mood to euphoric or dysphoric states (or both) beyond normal mood shifts (as distinguished from Manic Thought/Behavior).

Motor Hyperactivity Movements and actions that are performed at a greater than normal rate of speed, as in an individual who is constantly restless and in motion (e.g., the hyperactive behaviors of children).

***Obsessions** Unwelcome ideas, emotions, or urges that repetitiously and insistently force themselves into consciousness.

Oppositionalism Pervasive disobedience, negativism, or provocative contrariness to adult authority figures.

Pathological Grief Unreasonable or extended bereavement following a loss.

Pathological Guilt Persistent feelings of guilt not justified by the reasons stated.

***Phobia** An irrational morbid fear of persons, places, or things.

***Physical Abuse Perpetrator** The perpetrator of deliberate physical acts (including physical neglect) that injure or may potentially injure a family member or significant other (as distinguished from Assaultiveness, Homicidal Thought/Behavior, and Sexual Trauma Perpetrator).

Physical Abuse Victim The victim of deliberate physical acts (including physical neglect) perpetrated by a family member or significant other (excludes Sexual Trauma Victim).

Promiscuity Engaging in indiscriminate casual sexual relations with a high frequency and many partners.

***Psychomotor Retardation** Slowness of response or thought process and decrease in motor activity.

***Psychotic Thought/Behavior** Marked illogicality or peculiar ideation, derailment or loosening of associations, poverty of thought, and grossly disorganized behaviors that may be dangerous or unexplainable.

***Running Away** Reckless or planned elopements from home without parental authorization.

School Avoidance Persistent reluctance or refusal to attend school to stay with major attachment figures or remain at home.

Self-Esteem Deficiency Inadequate or absent regard for oneself; includes hypersensitivity to criticism in individuals not manifestly dysphoric.

***Self-Mutilation** Maiming or injuring one's body, such as cutting or hair pulling; this includes willful production of any symptom, syndrome, or disease (Münchhausen Syndrome) (excludes Suicidal Thought/Behavior).

Sexual Object Choice Dysfunction Sexual urges or behaviors that are distressing, harmful, or dangerous to the patient or others (as distinguished from Sexual Trauma Perpetrator).

Sexual Performance Dysfunction Altered sexual arousal, desire, or performance.

***Sexual Trauma Perpetrator** The perpetrator of sexual molestation or rape (as distinguished from Assaultiveness and Sexual Object Choice Dysfunction).

Sexual Trauma Victim The victim of sexual molestation or rape.

Social Withdrawal Curtailment or cessation of interpersonal relationships to an extent that interferes with the ability to function adequately.

Somatization Organic expression of psychological disturbances.

Stealing Repeated violation of the rights and property of others, including taking what belongs to others.

*__Substance Abuse__ Continued use of a mood-altering substance despite the obvious social, occupational, psychological, or physical problems caused by the use of psychoactive substances.

*__Suicidal Thought/Behavior__ Thoughts of or attempts at killing oneself.

Tantrums Dramatic outbursts of crying, kicking, or screaming in response to frustration; may include holding the breath, biting, cursing, head banging, striking people, and throwing things (as distinguished from Assaultiveness).

Truancy Unauthorized absence from school or work.

Uncommunicativeness Unwillingness or inability to impart information, thoughts, or feelings to others.

Uncontrolled Buying Persistent or excessive purchasing with real or potential risk to the patient or others.

Uncontrolled Gambling Persistent or excessive participation in games of chance with real or potential risk to the patient or others.

Appendix B

Severity Rating Qualifiers (Critical Impairments)

Critical impairments comprise a select subgroup of impairments that have the potential to require more service-intensive treatment, a more intensive treatment setting, or acute care. Although all the impairments can be rated with a severity 1 or 2, the critical impairments listed may also manifest with a severity 3 or 4. There are actually five severity ratings, including a rating of 0; there are no qualifiers for a 0 rating of an impairment:

Severity 4: Imminently Dangerous
Severity 3: Severely Incapacitating
Severity 2: Destabilizing
Severity 1: Distressing
Severity 0: Absent or Nonpathological

Anxiety

Severity 4:

Places self or others in immediate, life-threatening danger.
Present > 75% of the day.
Totally interferes (> 90%) with the ability to care for oneself.
Totally interferes (> 90%) with:
carrying out daily personal, family, financial, or legal responsibilities, or
following a prescribed treatment regimen.

Patient unaware of the life-threatening consequences of the unremitting Anxiety.

Severity 3:

Places self or others in likely danger.

Present > 50% of the day.

Severely interferes (65%–90%) with:

carrying out daily personal, family, financial, or legal responsibilities,

or

performing complex/new tasks at work/school,

or

following a prescribed treatment regimen.

Patient unable to interrupt or reduce the Anxiety.

Severity 2:

Present > 25% of the day.

More than two episodes per day.

Markedly interferes (30%–60%) with:

carrying out personal, family, financial, or legal responsibilities,

or

performing complex/new tasks at work/school,

or

following a prescribed treatment regimen.

Markedly disruptive (> 30%) to the daily functioning of others.

Adequate reduction of Anxiety requires intensive therapeutic support.

Severity 1:

Present daily to weekly.

Compromises (< 30%) optimal ability to:

carry out daily personal, family, financial, or legal responsibilities,

or

perform complex/new tasks at work/school,

or

follow a prescribed treatment regimen.

Compromises (< 30%) the optimal daily functioning of others.

Adequate management of the Anxiety requires frequent therapeutic support.

Assaultiveness

Severity 4:

Places self or others in immediate, life-threatening danger.

Patient totally unable or unwilling to control Assaultiveness.

Present at least daily.

Recent history of dangerous Assaultiveness.

Severity 3:

Places self or others in likely danger.

Patient variably unable or unwilling to control Assaultiveness.

Present within the last week.

History of dangerous Assaultiveness.

Severity 2:

Assaultiveness threats present.

Patient variably able to control Assaultiveness.

History of Assaultiveness.

Markedly interferes (> 30%) with the daily functioning of others.

Severity 1:

Assaultive ideation present.

History of assaultive threats or ideation.

Compromises (< 30%) the optimal daily functioning of others.

Compulsions

Severity 4:

Places self or others in immediate, life-threatening danger.

Present multiple times daily.

Interruption of Compulsions increases Anxiety, further impairing ability to function.

Totally interferes (> 90%) with the ability to care for oneself.

Totally interferes (> 90%) with:

carrying out daily personal, family, financial, or legal responsibilities, or

following a prescribed treatment regimen.

Severity 3:

Places self or others in likely danger.

Present at least daily.

Patient totally unable to interrupt Compulsions.

Severely interferes (61%–90%) with the ability to care for oneself.

Severely interferes (61%–90%) with:

carrying out daily personal, family, financial, or legal responsibilities,

or

performing complex/new tasks at work/school,

or

following a prescribed treatment regimen.

Severity 2:

Present daily to weekly.

Patient can interrupt the Compulsions only with intensive therapeutic support.

Markedly interferes (30%–60%) with the ability to care for oneself.

Markedly interferes (30%–60%) with:

carrying out daily personal, family, financial, or legal responsibilities,

or

performing complex/new tasks at work/school,

or

following a prescribed treatment regimen.

Markedly disruptive (> 30%) to the daily functioning of others.

Severity 1:

Patient can interrupt the Compulsions only with frequent therapeutic support.

Compromises (< 30%) optimal ability to care for oneself.

Compromises (< 30%) optimal ability to:

carry out daily personal, family, financial, or legal responsibilities,

or

perform complex/new tasks at work/school,

or

follow a prescribed treatment regimen.

Compromises (< 30%) the optimal daily functioning of others.

Concomitant Medical Condition

Severity 4:

Life threatening for the patient.

Patient totally unable or unwilling to manage the Concomitant Medical Condition.

Totally interferes (> 90%) with the ability to care for oneself.

Severity 3:

Dangerous but not imminently life threatening for the patient.

Patient denies extent of the Concomitant Medical Condition.

Patient denies potential dangerous consequences of inadequate management of the Concomitant Medical Condition.

Severity 2:

Concomitant Medical Condition is unstable.

Patient management of the Concomitant Medical Condition is medically unacceptable.

Severity 1:

Concomitant Medical Condition requires regular medical supervision.

Patient verbalizes distress about the presence of the Concomitant Medical Condition.

Delusions (Nonparanoid)

Severity 4:

Places self or others in immediate, life-threatening danger.

Unremitting delusional thinking.

Patient convinced Delusions are true and acts accordingly.

Totally interferes (> 90%) with the ability to care for oneself.

Totally interferes (> 90%) with:

carrying out daily personal, family, financial, or legal responsibilities,

or

following a prescribed treatment regimen.

Confrontation about the Delusions increases Anxiety, further impairing ability to function.

Severity 3:

Places self or others in likely danger.

Preoccupation with Delusions at least half the time.

Patient believes Delusions are true but does not act on them.

Severely interferes (61%–90%) with the ability to care for oneself.

Severely interferes (61%–90%) with:

carrying out daily personal, family, financial, or legal responsibilities,

or

performing complex/new tasks at work/school,

or

following a prescribed treatment regimen.

Severity 2:

Patient unsure if Delusions are true.

Present daily to weekly.

Markedly interferes (30%–60%) with the ability to care for oneself.

Markedly interferes (30%–60%) with:

carrying out daily personal, family, financial, or legal responsibilities,

or

performing complex/new tasks at work/school,

or

following a prescribed treatment regimen.

Markedly disruptive (> 30%) to the daily functioning of others.

Severity 1:

Patient able to consider alternative explanations for delusional thinking.

Compromises (< 30%) optimal ability to care for oneself.

Compromises (< 30%) optimal ability to:

carry out daily personal, family, financial, or legal responsibilities,

or

perform complex/new tasks at work/school,

or

follow a prescribed treatment regimen.

Compromises (> 30%) the optimal daily functioning of others.

Delusions (Paranoid)

Severity 4:

Places self or others in immediate, life-threatening danger.

Unremitting paranoid thinking.

Patient convinced paranoid beliefs are true and acts accordingly.

Totally interferes (> 90%) with the ability to care for oneself.

Totally interferes (< 90%) with:

carrying out daily personal, family, financial, or legal responsibilities,

or

following a prescribed treatment regimen.

Confrontation about the paranoid thinking increases Anxiety, further impairing ability to function.

Severity 3:

Places self or others in likely danger.

Preoccupation with paranoid beliefs at least half the time.

Patient believes delusions are true but does not act on them.
Severely interferes (61%–90%) with the ability to care for oneself.
Severely interferes (61%–90%) with:
carrying out daily personal, family, financial, or legal responsibilities,
or
performing complex/new tasks at work/school,
or
following a prescribed treatment regimen.

Severity 2:
Patient unsure if paranoid beliefs are true.
Present daily to weekly.
Markedly interferes (30%–60%) with the ability to care for oneself.
Markedly interferes (30%–60%) with:
carrying out daily personal, family, financial, or legal responsibilities,
or
performing complex/new tasks at work/school,
or
following a prescribed treatment regimen.
Markedly disruptive (> 30%) to the daily functioning of others.

Severity 1:
Patient able to consider alternative explanations for delusional thinking.
Compromises (< 30%) optimal ability to care for oneself.
Compromises (< 30%) optimal ability to:
carry out daily personal, family, financial, or legal responsibilities,
or
perform complex/new tasks at work/school,
or
follow a prescribed treatment regimen.
Compromises (> 30%) the optimal daily functioning of others.

Dissociative States

Severity 4:
Places self or others in immediate, life-threatening danger.
Patient totally unaware of the presence of Dissociative States.
Present daily.
Totally interferes (> 90%) with the ability to care for oneself.

Totally interferes (> 90%) with:

carrying out daily personal, family, financial, or legal responsibilities,

or

following a prescribed treatment regimen.

Severity 3:

Places self or others in likely danger.

Patient totally unable to control the Dissociative States.

Present at least weekly.

Severely interferes (61%–90%) with the ability to care for oneself.

Severely interferes (61%–90%) with:

carrying out daily personal, family, financial, or legal responsibilities,

or

performing complex/new tasks at work/school,

or

following a prescribed treatment regimen.

Severity 2:

Dissociative States present with a previous history of Dissociative States.

Markedly interferes (30%–60%) with the ability to care for oneself.

Markedly interferes (30%–60%) with:

carrying out daily personal, family, financial, or legal responsibilities,

or

performing complex/new tasks at work/school,

or

following a prescribed treatment regimen.

Patient can interrupt the Dissociative States only with intensive therapeutic support.

Markedly disruptive (> 30%) to the daily functioning of others.

Severity 1:

Patient verbalizes fear that previously experienced Dissociative States will recur.

Compromises (< 30%) optimal ability to care for oneself.

Compromises (< 30%) optimal ability to:

carry out daily personal, family, financial, or legal responsibilities,

or

perform complex/new tasks at work/school,

or

follow a prescribed treatment regimen.

Patient can interrupt the Dissociative States only with frequent therapeutic support.
Compromises (< 30%) the optimal daily functioning of others.

Dysphoric Mood

Severity 4:
Places self or others in immediate, life-threatening danger.
Present > 75% of the day.
Totally interferes (> 90%) with the ability to care for oneself.
Totally interferes (> 90%) with:
carrying out daily personal, family, financial, or legal responsibilities,
or
following a prescribed treatment regimen.

Severity 3:
Places self or others in likely danger.
Severely interferes (61%–90%) with the ability to care for oneself.
Severely interferes (61%–90%) with:
carrying out daily personal, family, financial, or legal responsibilities,
or
performing complex/new tasks at work/school,
or
following a prescribed treatment regimen.

Severity 2:
Present > 25% of the day.
Markedly interferes (30%–60%) with the ability to care for oneself.
Markedly interferes (30%–60%) with:
carrying out daily personal, family, financial, or legal responsibilities,
or
performing complex/new tasks at work/school,
or
following a prescribed treatment regimen.
Patient requires intensive therapeutic support to interrupt the Dysphoric Mood.

Severity 1:
Present daily to weekly.
Compromises (< 30%) optimal ability to care for oneself.
Compromises (< 30%) optimal ability to:

carry out daily personal, family, financial, or legal responsibilities,

or

perform complex/new tasks at work/school,

or

follow a prescribed treatment regimen.

Patient requires frequent therapeutic support to interrupt Dysphoric Mood.

Eating Disorder

Severity 4:

Places self in immediate, life-threatening danger.

Patient unaware of the presence of an Eating Disorder.

Symptoms present multiple times daily.

Patient has psychotic distortion of body image.

Totally interferes (> 90%) with the ability to care for oneself.

Severity 3:

Places self in likely danger.

Patient is totally unable to control Eating Disorder symptoms.

Symptoms present daily.

Patient has severely distorted body image.

Severely interferes (61%–90%) with the ability to care for oneself.

Severely interferes (61%–90%) with:

carrying out daily personal, family, financial, or legal responsibilities,

or

performing complex/new tasks at work/school,

or

following a prescribed treatment regimen.

Severity 2:

Symptoms present at least weekly.

Markedly interferes (30%–60%) with the ability to care for oneself.

Markedly interferes (30%–60%) with:

carrying out daily personal, family, financial, or legal responsibilities,

or

performing complex/new tasks at work/school,

or

following a prescribed treatment regimen.

Patient can interrupt the Eating Disorder symptoms only with intensive therapeutic support.

Severity 1:

Compromises (< 30%) optimal ability to care for oneself.

Compromises (< 30%) optimal ability to:

carry out daily personal, family, financial, or legal responsibilities,

or

perform complex/new tasks at work/school,

or

follow a prescribed treatment regimen.

Patient can interrupt the Eating Disorder symptoms only with frequent therapeutic support.

Fire Setting

Severity 4:

Places self or others in immediate, life-threatening danger.

Patient has active plans or threats to set a fire.

Repeated past history of Fire Setting.

Severity 3:

Places self or others in likely danger.

Patient is totally unable to interrupt Fire-Setting plans.

Patient has a recent history of setting a fire.

Recent history of planning or securing the means to set a fire.

Severity 2:

Markedly interferes (> 30%) with the daily functioning of self or others.

Patient has frequent Fire-Setting preoccupations.

Patient can interrupt setting a fire or planning to set a fire only with intensive therapeutic support.

Severity 1:

Compromises (< 30%) the daily functioning of self or others.

History of Fire-Setting ideation.

Patient can interrupt Fire-Setting plans only with frequent therapeutic support.

Hallucinations

Severity 4:

Places self or others in immediate, life-threatening danger.

Patient has unremitting Hallucinations.

Patient convinced Hallucinations are real and acts accordingly.

Totally interferes (> 90%) with the ability to care for oneself.

Totally interferes (> 90%) with:

carrying out daily personal, family, financial, or legal responsibilities, or

following a prescribed treatment regimen.

Confrontation about the Hallucinations increases Anxiety, further impairing ability to function.

Severity 3:

Places self or others in likely danger.

Patient is preoccupied with Hallucinations at least half the time.

Patient believes or is reasonably sure that Hallucinations are real but does not act on them.

Severely interferes (61%–90%) with the ability to care for oneself.

Severely interferes (61%–90%) with:

carrying out daily personal, family, financial, or legal responsibilities, or

performing complex/new tasks at work/school,

or

following a prescribed treatment regimen.

Severely disruptive (61%–90%) to the daily functioning of others.

Severity 2:

Patient unsure if Hallucinations are real.

Present daily to weekly.

Markedly interferes (30%–60%) with the ability to care for oneself.

Markedly interferes (30%–60%) with:

carrying out daily personal, family, financial, or legal responsibilities, or

performing complex/new tasks at work/school,

or

following a prescribed treatment regimen.

Markedly disruptive (30%–60%) to the daily functioning of others.

Severity 1:

Hallucinations present, but patient acknowledges they are not real.

Compromises (< 30%) optimal ability to care for oneself.

Compromises (< 30%) optimal ability to:

carry out daily personal, family, financial, or legal responsibilities, or

follow a prescribed treatment regimen.

Compromises (< 30%) the optimal daily functioning of others.

Homicidal Thought/Behavior

Severity 4:

Places self or others in immediate, life-threatening danger.

Patient demonstrates no concern for the consequences of Homicidal Thought/Behavior.

Patient has a recent history of Homicidal Behavior.

Severity 3:

Places self or others in likely danger.

Patient is unable to interrupt Homicidal Behavior.

Patient has a past history of Homicidal Behavior.

Severity 2:

Patient is unable to state convincingly that Homicidal Thoughts will not lead to action.

Recent history of homicidal threats.

Markedly interferes (> 30%) with the daily functioning of others.

Severity 1:

Homicidal Thoughts present with verbalized confidence that they will not be acted on.

Past history of homicidal threats.

Compromises (< 30%) the daily functioning of others.

Inadequate Healthcare Skills

Severity 4:

Places self in immediate, life-threatening danger.

Patient totally unaware of the life-threatening consequences of Inadequate Healthcare Skills.

Totally interferes (> 90%) with the ability to care for oneself.

Totally interferes (> 90%) with:

carrying out daily personal, family, financial, or legal responsibilities,
or
following a prescribed treatment regimen.

Severity 3:

Places self in likely danger.
Patient unable to improve the Inadequate Healthcare Skills that may be a danger to oneself.
Severely interferes (61%–90%) with the ability to care for oneself.
Severely interferes (61%–90%) with:
carrying out daily personal, family, financial, or legal responsibilities,
or
performing complex/new tasks at work/school,
or
following a prescribed treatment regimen.

Severity 2:

Improvement of the Inadequate Healthcare Skills requires intensive therapeutic support.
Markedly interferes (30%–60%) with the ability to care for oneself.
Markedly interferes (30%–60%) with:
carrying out daily personal, family, financial, or legal responsibilities,
or
performing complex/new tasks at work/school,
or
following a prescribed treatment regimen.

Severity 1:

Improvement of Inadequate Healthcare Skills requires frequent therapeutic support.
Compromises (< 30%) optimal ability to care for oneself.
Compromises (< 30%) optimal ability to:
carry out daily personal, family, financial, or legal responsibilities,
or
perform complex/new tasks at work/school,
or
follow a prescribed treatment regimen.

Manic Thought/Behavior

Severity 4:

Places self or others in immediate, life-threatening danger.

Totally interferes (> 90%) with the ability to care for oneself.

Totally interferes (> 90%) with:

- carrying out daily personal, family, financial, or legal responsibilities,
- or
- following a prescribed treatment regimen.

Confrontation about the Manic Thought/Behavior increases Anxiety, further impairing ability to function.

Severity 3:

Places self or others in likely danger.

Severely interferes (61%–90%) with the ability to care for oneself.

Severely interferes (61%–90%) with:

- carrying out daily personal, family, financial, or legal responsibilities,
- or
- performing complex/new tasks at work/school,
- or
- following a prescribed treatment regimen.

Severity 2:

Markedly interferes (30%–60%) with the ability to care for oneself.

Markedly interferes (30%–60%) with:

- carrying out daily personal, family, financial, or legal responsibilities,
- or
- performing complex/new tasks at work/school,
- or
- following a prescribed treatment regimen.

Markedly disruptive (> 30%) to the daily functioning of others.

Severity 1:

Compromises (< 30%) optimal ability to care for oneself.

Compromises (< 30%) optimal ability to:

- carry out daily personal, family, financial, or legal responsibilities,
- or
- perform complex/new tasks at work/school,
- or
- follow a prescribed treatment regimen.

Compromises (< 30%) the optimal daily functioning of others.

Medical Risk Factor

Severity 4:

Requires 24-hour intensive care unit (ICU) monitoring.

Patient has a history of a life-threatening Medical Risk Factor.

Severity 3:

Requires 24-hour inpatient monitoring.

Patient has a history of a potentially life-threatening Medical Risk Factor.

Severity 2:

Requires daily medical monitoring.

Patient has a history of a dangerous Medical Risk Factor.

Severity 1:

Requires regular frequent monitoring.

Patient has a history of a Medical Risk Factor.

Mood Lability

Severity 4:

Places self or others in immediate, life-threatening danger.

Totally interferes (> 90%) with the ability to care for oneself.

Totally interferes (> 90%) with:

carrying out daily personal, family, financial, or legal responsibilities,

or

following a prescribed treatment regimen.

Severity 3:

Places self or others in likely danger.

Severely interferes (61%–90%) with the ability to care for oneself.

Severely interferes (61%–90%) with:

carrying out daily personal, family, financial, or legal responsibilities,

or

performing complex/new tasks at work/school,

or

following a prescribed treatment regimen.

Severity 2:

Markedly interferes (30%–60%) with the ability to care for oneself.

Markedly interferes (30%–60%) with:

carrying out daily personal, family, financial, or legal responsibilities,

or

performing complex/new tasks at work/school,
or
following a prescribed treatment regimen.
Markedly disruptive (> 30%) to the daily functioning of others.

Severity 1:

Compromises (< 30%) optimal ability to care for oneself.
Compromises (< 30%) optimal ability to:
carry out daily personal, family, financial, or legal responsibilities,
or
perform complex/new tasks at work/school,
or
follow a prescribed treatment regimen.
Compromises (> 30%) the optimal daily functioning of others.

Obsessions

Severity 4:

Places self or others in immediate, life-threatening danger.
Present multiple times daily.
Interruption of the Obsessions increases Anxiety, further impairing ability to function.
Totally interferes (> 90%) with the ability to care for oneself.
Totally interferes (> 90%) with:
carrying out daily personal, family, financial, or legal responsibilities,
or
following a prescribed treatment regimen.

Severity 3:

Places self or others in likely danger.
Present at least daily.
Patient is totally unable to interrupt the Obsessions.
Severely interferes (61%–90%) with the ability to care for oneself.
Severely interferes (61%–90%) with:
carrying out daily personal, family, financial, or legal responsibilities,
or
performing complex/new tasks at work/school,
or
following a prescribed treatment regimen.

Severity 2:

Present daily to weekly.

Patient can interrupt the Obsessions only with intensive therapeutic support.

Markedly interferes (30%–60%) with the ability to care for oneself.

Markedly interferes (30%–60%) with:

carrying out daily personal, family, financial, or legal responsibilities,

or

performing complex/new tasks at work/school,

or

following a prescribed treatment regimen.

Markedly disruptive (> 30%) to the functioning of others.

Severity 1:

Patient able to interrupt the Obsessions only with frequent therapeutic support.

Compromises (< 30%) optimal ability to care for oneself.

Compromises (< 30%) optimal ability to:

carry out daily personal, family, financial, or legal responsibilities,

or

perform complex/new tasks at work/school,

or

follow a prescribed treatment regimen.

Compromises (< 30%) the optimal daily functioning of self or others.

Phobia

Severity 4:

Places self or others in immediate, life-threatening danger.

Forced encounter with the phobic object or situation increases Anxiety, further impairing ability to function.

Totally interferes (> 90%) with the ability to care for oneself.

Totally interferes (> 90%) with:

carrying out daily personal, family, financial, or legal responsibilities,

or

following a prescribed treatment regimen.

Severity 3:

Places self or others in likely danger.

Patient is totally unable to confront the phobic object or situation.

Severely interferes (61%–90%) with the ability to care for oneself.
Severely interferes (61%–90%) with:
carrying out daily personal, family, financial, or legal responsibilities,
or
performing complex/new tasks at work/school,
or
following a prescribed treatment regimen.

Severity 2:

Patient is able to encounter the phobic object or situation only with intensive therapeutic support.
Markedly interferes (30%–60%) with the ability to care for oneself.
Markedly interferes (30%–60%) with:
carrying out daily personal, family, financial, or legal responsibilities,
or
performing complex/new tasks at work/school,
or
following a prescribed treatment regimen.
Markedly disruptive (> 30%) to the functioning of others.

Severity 1:

Patient is able to encounter the phobic object or situation only with frequent therapeutic support.
Compromises (< 30%) optimal ability to care for oneself.
Compromises (< 30%) optimal ability to:
carry out daily personal, family, financial, or legal responsibilities,
or
perform complex/new tasks at work/school,
or
follow a prescribed treatment regimen.
Compromises (< 30%) the optimal daily functioning of others.

Physical Abuse Perpetrator

Severity 4:

Places others in immediate, life-threatening danger.
Patient is totally unable to control physically abusive behavior.
Patient is currently being investigated or charged for perpetrating life-threatening physical abuse.
Patient has a recent history of very violent responses to minimal frustration.

Severity 3:

Places others in likely danger.

Patient is unable to interrupt the physically abusive behavior.

Patient has been recently or repeatedly reported to the appropriate public agency or law officials for the dangerous physically abusive behavior.

Patient has a history of violent responses to frustration.

Severity 2:

Patient is only variably able to interrupt the physically abusive behavior.

Patient has a history of physically abusive behavior.

Severity 1:

Patient is unable to interrupt making threats of physical abuse.

Patient verbalizes concern about being able to always contain physically abusive behavior.

Psychomotor Retardation

Severity 4:

Places self or others in immediate, life-threatening danger.

Constant and persistent Psychomotor Retardation.

Totally interferes (> 90%) with the ability to care for oneself.

Totally interferes (> 90%) with:

carrying out daily personal, family, financial, or legal responsibilities,

or

following a prescribed treatment regimen.

Patient is totally unaware of the life-threatening Psychomotor Retardation.

Severity 3:

Places self or others in likely danger.

Present > 50% of the day.

Severely interferes (61%–90%) with the ability to care for oneself.

Severely interferes (61%–90%) with:

carrying out daily personal, family, financial, or legal responsibilities,

or

performing complex/new tasks at work/school,

or

following a prescribed treatment regimen.

Patient is unable to initiate any cognitive or behavioral activity.

Severity 2:

Periods of Psychomotor Retardation present daily.

Markedly interferes (30%–60%) with the ability to care for oneself.

Markedly interferes (30%–60%) with:

carrying out daily personal, family, financial, or legal responsibilities,

or

performing complex/new tasks at work/school,

or

following a prescribed treatment regimen.

Patient is unable to initiate cognitive or behavioral activity without intensive therapeutic support.

Markedly disruptive (> 30%) to the daily functioning of others.

Severity 1:

Psychomotor Retardation present for a period of the day at least weekly.

Compromises (< 30%) optimal ability to care for oneself.

Compromises (< 30%) optimal ability to:

carry out daily personal, family, financial, or legal responsibilities,

or

perform complex/new tasks at work/school,

or

follow a prescribed treatment regimen.

Patient is unable to initiate cognitive or behavioral activity without frequent therapeutic support.

Compromises (< 30%) the optimal daily functioning of others.

Psychotic Thought/Behavior

Severity 4:

Places self or others in immediate, life-threatening danger.

Confronting the patient's Psychotic Thought/Behavior increases psychotic agitation.

Totally interferes (> 90%) with:

carrying out daily personal, family, financial, or legal responsibilities,

or

following a prescribed treatment regimen.

Severity 3:

Places self or others in likely danger.

Patient is unable to consider that the Psychotic Thoughts are unreal.

Severely interferes (61%–90%) with the ability to care for oneself.

Severely interferes (61%–90%) with:

carrying out daily personal, family, financial, or legal responsibilities, or

performing complex/new tasks at work/school,

or

following a prescribed treatment regimen.

Severity 2:

Patient is unsure if Psychotic Thought is real.

Markedly interferes (30%–60%) with the ability to care for oneself.

Markedly interferes (30%–60%) with:

carrying out daily personal, family, financial, or legal responsibilities, or

performing complex/new tasks at work/school,

or

following a prescribed treatment regimen.

Markedly disruptive (> 30%) to the daily functioning of others.

Severity 1:

Patient is not always able to differentiate Psychotic from Nonpsychotic Thought.

Compromises (< 30%) optimal ability to care for oneself.

Compromises (< 30%) optimal ability to:

carry out daily personal, family, financial, or legal responsibilities, or

perform complex/new tasks at work/school,

or

follow a prescribed treatment regimen.

Compromises (< 30%) the optimal daily functioning of others.

Running Away

Severity 4:

Places self in immediate, life-threatening danger.

Multiple runaway attempts.

Patient shows no concern for the potential danger of Running Away.

Totally interferes (> 90%) with the ability to care for oneself.

Severity 3:

Places self in likely danger.

Runaway attempt or actively threatened to run away within the last week.

Severely interferes (61%–90%) with the ability to care for oneself.

Severity 2:

Patient is totally unable to control the urge to run away.

Recent attempts to run away or recent threats of Running Away.

Markedly interferes (30%–60%) with the ability to care for oneself.

Severity 1:

Persistent thoughts of Running Away.

Compromises (< 30%) optimal ability to care for oneself.

Self-Mutilation

Severity 4:

Places self in immediate, life-threatening danger.

Patient persists with attempts at Self-Mutilation with no demonstrable intent or ability to stop.

Attempts by others to interrupt the Self-Mutilation only increase Anxiety and further impair the ability to function.

Totally interferes (> 90%) with the ability to care for oneself.

Totally interferes (> 90%) with:

carrying out daily personal, family, financial, or legal responsibilities, or

following a prescribed treatment regimen.

Severity 3:

Places self in likely danger.

Patient unable to interrupt Self-Mutilation behavior.

Severely interferes (61%–90%) with the ability to care for oneself.

Severely interferes (61%–90%) with:

carrying out daily personal, family, financial, or legal responsibilities, or

following a prescribed treatment regimen.

Severity 2:

Frequent Self-Mutilation ideation with a recent history of Self-Mutilation.

Patient can interrupt Self-Mutilation only with intensive therapeutic support.

Markedly interferes (30%–60%) with the ability to care for oneself.

Markedly interferes (30%–60%) with:

carrying out daily personal, family, financial, or legal responsibilities.

Severity 1:

Patient can interrupt Self-Mutilation thoughts or behaviors only with frequent therapeutic support.

Compromises (< 30%) optimal ability to care for oneself.

Compromises (< 30%) optimal ability to:

carry out daily personal, family, financial, or legal responsibilities.

Sexual Trauma Perpetrator

Severity 4:

Places others in immediate, life-threatening danger.

Patient is totally unable to control rape or molestation behaviors.

Patient is currently charged or recently convicted of a rape or molestation crime.

Severity 3:

Places others in likely danger.

Patient is unable to interrupt the urge to rape or molest another person.

Patient has been recently or repeatedly charged with a rape or molestation crime.

Severity 2:

Patient is unable to interrupt rape or molestation ideation.

Patient has a criminal record of rape or molestation charges.

Severity 1:

Patient verbalizes fear and concern that ideas of molesting or raping another person are not under control.

Patient has a history of rape or molestation ideation.

Substance Abuse

Severity 4:

Places self or others in immediate, life-threatening danger.

Patient has been abusing substances for at least 4 weeks—cessation of which places the patient at high risk for a life-threatening physical withdrawal syndrome.

Totally interferes (> 90%) with the ability to care for oneself.

Totally interferes (> 90%) with:

carrying out daily personal, family, financial, or legal responsibilities,

or

following a prescribed treatment regimen.

Patient has a history of one or more episodes of life-threatening alcohol or drug withdrawal.

Patient has a Concomitant Medical Condition that is imminently dangerous (severity 4).

Patient has another impairment that is imminently dangerous (severity 4).

Severity 3:

Places self or others in likely danger.

Patient has been abusing substances for the last 4 weeks—cessation of which places the patient at risk for withdrawal.

Patient is unable to maintain abstinence for 24 hours without around-the-clock supervision.

Severely interferes (> 90%) with the ability to care for oneself.

Severely interferes (61%–90%) with:

carrying out daily personal, family, financial, or legal responsibilities,

or

performing complex/new tasks at work/school,

or

following a prescribed treatment regimen.

Patient has a history of two or more failures of detoxification at less intensive levels of care.

Patient has a Concomitant Medical Condition that is incapacitating (severity 3).

Patient has another psychiatric impairment that is incapacitating (severity 3).

Patient's previous efforts to maintain abstinence have been actively sabotaged by either:

family or significant other,

or

occupation or social setting.

Severity 2:

Patient is unable to maintain abstinence while participating in a treatment program for more than 3 months without relapsing.

Patient is unable to maintain abstinence for more than 3 months following completion of an outpatient program.

Markedly interferes (30%–60%) with:

carrying out daily personal, family, financial, or legal responsibilities,

or

performing complex/new tasks at work/school,

or

following a prescribed treatment regimen.

Patient has a Concomitant Medical Condition that is destabilizing (severity 2).

Patient has another psychiatric impairment that is destabilizing (severity 2).

Patient's current treatment is likely to be interfered with or potentially sabotaged by either:

family or significant other,

or

occupation or social setting.

Severity 1:

Patient requires regular therapeutic support to maintain abstinence.

Compromises (< 30%) optimal ability to:

carry out daily personal, family, financial, or legal responsibilities,

or

perform complex/new tasks at work/school,

or

follow a prescribed treatment regimen.

Patient has a Concomitant Medical Condition that is distressing (severity 1).

Patient has another psychiatric impairment that is distressing (severity 1).

Compromises the optimal daily functioning of others.

Suicidal Thought/Behavior

Severity 4:

Places self in immediate, life-threatening danger.

Patient has unremitting intent to commit suicide.

Patient has made a recent life-threatening suicide attempt.

Patient actively plans lethal suicide attempts at least daily.

Totally interferes (> 90%) with the ability to care for oneself.

Severity 3:

Places self or others in likely danger.

Patient has active suicide plans that are prevented up to 8 hours using a signed agreement to that effect.

Recent history of dangerous suicide attempt.

Active suicide plans or suicide gestures daily.

Severely interferes (61%–90%) with the ability to care for oneself.

Severity 2:

Suicide ideation or plan present at least weekly.

Patient has active suicide plans that are prevented up to 24 hours using a signed agreement to that effect.

Past history (> 3 months ago) of suicide attempt or recent history of active suicide plans.

Patient can interrupt Suicidal Thought/Behavior only with intensive therapeutic support.

Severity 1:

Suicide ideation present.

Patient has a history of one or more suicide gestures or nonlethal attempts.

Patient can interrupt Suicidal Thought/Behavior only with frequent therapeutic support.

Appendix C

Patient Objectives Reference List (Critical Impairments)

* *Note to the reader: The patient objectives listed for these impairments are intended to be suggestions only. These objectives are not a criteria set or the standardized treatment expectations for all patients, nor are these patient objectives the only ones relevant for a patient's treatment. Practitioners are encouraged to create additional patient objectives when needed. We do advise, however, that any new patient objectives adhere to the "patient will verbalize—patient will demonstrate" format utilized.*

Anxiety

Patient will verbalize:

Acceptance of responsibility for the presence of the Anxiety.

The precipitants for the Anxiety.

Understanding of the reasons for the Anxiety.

Warning signs that the Anxiety is exacerbating.

A plan of action to be taken should the Anxiety exacerbate.

Patient will demonstrate:

Adherence to the medical treatment of the Anxiety.

Successful utilization of techniques such as autorelaxation or biofeedback to reduce the Anxiety.

Adequate management of the Anxiety.

Elimination of the Anxiety.

A completed self-care (discharge) plan, including steps to be taken should the Anxiety return or exacerbate.

Assaultiveness

Patient will verbalize:

Acceptance of responsibility for the Assaultiveness.

The recognized dangers of the Assaultiveness.

The adverse consequences of assaultive behaviors.

Alternative behaviors for Assaultiveness.

Warning signs that the Assaultiveness is exacerbating.

A plan of action to be taken should the Assaultiveness exacerbate.

Patient will demonstrate:

Participation in a prescribed treatment program.

Management of the Assaultiveness without the use of seclusion or restraints.

The capacity to verbalize anger rather than act on it.

Interruption of assaultive behavior before it occurs.

Elimination of assaultive behavior.

A completed self-care (discharge) plan, including steps to be taken should the Assaultiveness return or exacerbate.

Compulsions

Patient will verbalize:

Acceptance of the maladaptive consequences of the Compulsions.

The precipitants for the Compulsions.

Warning signs that the Compulsions are exacerbating.

A plan of action to be taken should the Compulsions exacerbate.

Patient will demonstrate:

Participation in a prescribed treatment program.

Adherence to the prescribed medication treatment program for the Compulsions.

Utilization of a behavior management program to reduce the Compulsions.

Adequate management of the Compulsions as evidenced by return of optimal daily functioning.

Elimination of the Compulsions.

A completed self-care (discharge) plan, including steps to be taken should the Compulsions return or exacerbate.

Concomitant Medical Condition

Patient will verbalize:

Acceptance of responsibility for management of the Concomitant Medical Condition.

Thoughts and feelings regarding the Concomitant Medical Condition.

Warning signs that the Concomitant Medical Condition is exacerbating.

A plan of action to be taken should the Concomitant Medical condition exacerbate.

Patient will demonstrate:

A self-care worksheet that describes the Concomitant Medical Condition, its etiology, prognosis, treatment regimen, and potential future complications.

Adherence to the treatment regimen for the Concomitant Medical Condition (e.g., self-initiated medication compliance, self-selected appropriate diet).

Adequate management of the Concomitant Medical Condition.

A completed self-care (discharge) plan, including steps to be taken should the Concomitant Medical Condition return or exacerbate.

Delusions (Nonparanoid)

Patient will verbalize:

Awareness of the presence of delusional thinking.

Responsibility for the presence of the Delusions.

The precipitants for the delusional thinking.

Warning signs that the Delusions are exacerbating.

A plan of action to be taken should the Delusions exacerbate.

Patient will demonstrate:

Absence of Delusions for 72 hours.

Adherence to the medical treatment of the Delusions.

Adequate management of the Delusions.

Absence of delusional thinking.

A completed self-care (discharge) plan, including steps to be taken should the Delusions return or exacerbate.

Delusions (Paranoid)

Patient will verbalize:

Awareness of the presence of paranoid thinking.

Acceptance of responsibility for the presence of the Paranoid Delusions.

The precipitants for the paranoid thinking.

Alternative explanations to paranoid thoughts.

Warning signs that the Paranoid Delusions are exacerbating.

A plan of action to be taken should the Paranoid Delusions exacerbate.

Patient will demonstrate:

Absence of paranoid thoughts for 72 hours.

Adherence to the medical treatment of the paranoid thinking.

Ability to "consider the alternative" thinking to paranoid thinking.

Adequate management of the paranoid thinking.

Absence of paranoid thinking.

A completed self-care (discharge) plan, including steps to be taken should the Paranoid Delusions return or exacerbate.

Dissociative States

Patient will verbalize:

Acceptance and responsibility for the presence of Dissociative States.

The maladaptive consequences of the Dissociative States.

The precipitants for the Dissociative States.
Warning signs that the Dissociative States are exacerbating.
A plan of action to be taken should the Dissociative States exacerbate.

Patient will demonstrate:

Adherence to the prescribed treatment program for the Dissociative States.
Utilization of behavior management program to eliminate Dissociative States for 72 hours.
Utilization of medication management program to eliminate Dissociative States for 72 hours.
Elimination of Dissociative States.
A completed self-care (discharge) plan, including steps to be taken should the Dissociative States return or exacerbate.

Dysphoric Mood

Patient will verbalize:

Acceptance of responsibility for the presence of the Dysphoric Mood.
Awareness of severe mood changes when they occur.
Awareness of the precipitants for negative mood changes and how to seek help accordingly.
Statements about self that are positive and hopeful rather than negative and self-deprecating.
Plans and activities to be initiated with family members or friends.
Warning signs that the Dysphoric Mood is exacerbating.
A plan of action to be taken should the Dysphoric Mood exacerbate.

Patient will demonstrate:

Reduction in the Dysphoric Mood as evidenced by a 50% decrease in the Hamilton Rating Scale for Depression (rated at the initiation of treatment) and/or a 50% improvement in the Coopersmith Self-Esteem Inventory.
Increased self-initiated and self-directed activities.
Increased integrating behaviors with others.
Elimination of isolative activities.
Participation in a prescribed treatment program.
Adherence to a medication management program.
Adequate management of the Dysphoric Mood as evidenced by patient report.

A completed self-care (discharge) plan, including steps to be taken should the Dysphoric Mood return or exacerbate.

Eating Disorder

Patient will verbalize:

Acceptance of a medically agreed-on ideal body weight.

The medical consequences of the abnormal eating behaviors.

The precipitants for aberrant eating behaviors.

Plans for the lifestyle changes necessary to maintain normal weight.

Absence of anxiety with respect to the established "normal" body weight.

Warning signs that the eating disorder is exacerbating.

A plan of action to be taken should the eating disorder exacerbate.

Patient will demonstrate:

Maintenance of daily "food intake log."

Maintenance for 1 week of at least 90% of expected body weight (in the case of anorexia/bulimia).

Maintenance of a 7-pound weight loss (in the case of overeating) for 1 week.

Maintenance of a medically agreed-on appropriate body weight with vital signs and laboratory studies within normal limits for 1 month.

Adherence to a prescribed treatment program for the Eating Disorder.

A completed self-care (discharge) plan, including steps to be taken should the Eating Disorder return or exacerbate.

Fire Setting

Patient will verbalize:

The dangerous consequences of the Fire Setting.

The precipitants for the Fire Setting.

Warning signs that the Fire Setting or urges to set fires are exacerbating.

A plan of action to be taken should the Fire Setting or urges to set fires exacerbate.

Patient will demonstrate:

Adherence to the prescribed treatment program for the Fire Setting.

Utilization of a behavior management program to eliminate Fire Setting.

Utilization of a medication management program to eliminate Fire Setting.

The ability to interrupt the urges to set fires.
Elimination of the Fire-Setting ideation/behaviors.
A completed self-care (discharge) plan, including steps to be taken should the Fire Setting or urges to set fires return or exacerbate.

Hallucinations

Patient will verbalize:

Awareness of the perceived sensory experiences as Hallucinations.
Acceptance of responsibility for the presence of the Hallucinations.
The precipitants for the Hallucinations.
Warning signs that the Hallucinations are exacerbating.
A plan of action to be taken should the Hallucinations exacerbate.

Patient will demonstrate:

Absence of Hallucinations for 72 hours.
Adherence to the medical treatment of the Hallucinations.
Adequate management of the Hallucinations.
Absence of Hallucinations.
A completed self-care (discharge) plan, including steps to be taken should the Hallucinations return or exacerbate.

Homicidal Thought/Behavior

Patient will verbalize:

Acceptance of responsibility for the Homicidal Thought/Behavior.
The adverse consequences of the Homicidal Thought/Behavior.
Alternative behaviors to interrupt Homicidal Thought/Behavior.
Warning signs that the Homicidal Thought/Behavior is exacerbating.
A plan of action to be taken should the Homicidal Thought/Behavior exacerbate.

Patient will demonstrate:

Adherence to a prescribed treatment program.
Verbalization of anger rather than acting on it.
Management of Homicidal Thought/Behavior without the use of seclusion or restraint for 72 hours.
Interruption of Homicidal Thought/Behavior before it occurs.
Elimination of active Homicidal Thought/Behavior.
A completed self-care (discharge) plan, including steps to be taken should the Homicidal Thought/Behavior return or exacerbate.

Inadequate Healthcare Skills

Patient will verbalize:

Acceptance of responsibility for the Inadequate Healthcare Skills.

Warning signs that the healthcare skills are deteriorating.

A plan of action to be taken should healthcare skills deteriorate.

Patient will demonstrate:

A self-care worksheet that describes the specific healthcare issues needing to be addressed.

The ability to bathe, brush teeth, comb hair, shave, and wear clean clothes daily.

The ability to select nutritious foods from the four food groups at mealtime.

Adherence to the treatment program for the Inadequate Healthcare Skills.

A completed self-care (discharge) plan, including steps to be taken should healthcare skills deteriorate.

Manic Thought/Behavior

Patient will verbalize:

Acceptance of responsibility for the presence of the Manic Thought/Behavior.

Awareness of Manic Thought/Behavior.

The precipitants for Manic Thought/Behavior.

Awareness of abrupt mood changes and how to ask for help accordingly.

Appropriate and reasonable plans to be initiated with family members or friends.

Warning signs that the Manic Thought/Behavior is exacerbating.

A plan of action to be taken should the Manic Thought/Behavior exacerbate.

Patient will demonstrate:

Reduction in Manic Thought/Behavior as evidenced by a 50% improvement in a mania assessment rating scale (rated at the initiation of treatment).

Reduction in Manic Thought/Behavior as evidenced by appropriate and reasonable statements about self and life.

Normalized self-directed initiation of activities.

Ability to spend one-half hour every shift in quiet and calm solitude.

Appropriate social interactions.

Adherence to a medication treatment program as evidenced by periodic blood testing of the prescribed drug to confirm therapeutic blood levels.

Adequate management of the Manic Thought/Behavior.

A completed self-care (discharge) plan, including steps to be taken should the Manic Thought/Behavior return or exacerbate.

Medical Risk Factor

Patient will verbalize:

Awareness of the presence and possible adverse consequences due to the Medical Risk Factor.

Understanding of the warning signs that the Medical Risk Factor is manifesting itself.

Patient will demonstrate:

Adherence to a treatment/monitoring program for the Medical Risk Factor.

Adequate and safe management of the Medical Risk Factor.

A completed self-care (discharge) plan, including steps to be taken should the Medical Risk Factor manifest in the future.

Medical Treatment Noncompliance

Patient will verbalize:

Acceptance of the need for long-term medical treatment compliance.

Thoughts and feelings regarding the Medical Treatment Noncompliance.

Warning signs that the Medical Treatment Noncompliance is exacerbating.

A plan of action to be taken should medical treatment compliance falter or deteriorate.

Patient will demonstrate:

A completed self-care worksheet that describes the potential risks, appropriate treatment regimen, and possible future complications of Medical Treatment Noncompliance.

Adherence to a prescribed medical treatment regimen.

A completed self-care (discharge) plan, including steps to be taken should medical treatment compliance falter or deteriorate.

Mood Lability

Patient will verbalize:

Awareness of the presence of the Mood Lability.

The precipitants for abrupt mood changes.

Warning signs that the Mood Lability is exacerbating.

A plan of action to be taken should the Mood Lability exacerbate.

Patient will demonstrate:

Adherence to a prescribed treatment program.

Seeking help from others when experiencing abrupt mood changes.

Consistent self-initiated activities when dysphoric.

Ability to regulate agitation and manic behavior individually.

Elimination of excessive isolation and/or overstimulating interactions with others.

Adherence to the medication treatment program as evidenced by periodic blood testing of the prescribed drug levels.

Adequate management of the Mood Lability.

A completed self-care (discharge) plan, including steps to be taken should the Mood Lability return or exacerbate.

Obsessions

Patient will verbalize:

Acceptance of the maladaptive consequences of the Obsessions.

The precipitants for the Obsessions.

Warning signs that the Obsessions are exacerbating.

A plan of action to be taken should the Obsessions exacerbate.

Patient will demonstrate:

Participation in a prescribed treatment program.

Adherence to the prescribed medication treatment program for the Obsessions.

Utilization of a behavior management program to reduce the Obsessions.

Adequate management of the Obsessions as evidenced by return of optimal daily functioning.

Elimination of the Obsessions.

A completed self-care (discharge) plan, including steps to be taken should the Obsessions return or exacerbate.

Phobia

Patient will verbalize:

Acceptance of the maladaptive consequences of the Phobia.

The precipitants for the Phobia.

Warning signs that the Phobia is exacerbating.

A plan of action to be taken should the Phobia exacerbate.

Patient will demonstrate:

Participation in a prescribed treatment program.

Adherence to the prescribed medication treatment program for the Phobia.

Utilization of a behavior management program to reduce the Phobia.

Adequate management of the phobia as evidenced by return of optimal daily functioning.

Elimination of the Phobia.

A completed self-care (discharge) plan, including steps to be taken should the Phobia return or exacerbate.

Physical Abuse Perpetrator

Patient will verbalize:

The dangers of physically abusive behaviors.

The damaging consequences of physically abusive behaviors.

Personal responsibility—rather than "blaming others"—for physically abusive behaviors.

A plan to avoid repeating physically abusive behaviors.

Alternative behaviors for being physically abusive.

Warning signs that urges to physically abuse are exacerbating.

A plan of action to be taken should urges to physically abuse exacerbate.

Patient will demonstrate:

Adherence to a prescribed treatment program.

The capacity to verbalize anger rather than act on it.

Elimination of the physically abusive behaviors.

A completed self-care (discharge) plan, including steps to be taken should the urges to physically abuse return or exacerbate.

Psychomotor Retardation

Patient will verbalize:

Acceptance of responsibility for the presence of the Psychomotor Retardation.

The precipitants for the Psychomotor Retardation.

The potential/real consequences of the Psychomotor Retardation.

Plans to be initiated with family members or friends.

Warning signs that the Psychomotor Retardation is exacerbating.

A plan of action to be taken should the Psychomotor Retardation exacerbate.

Patient will demonstrate:

Increased self-directed and self-initiated activities.

Increased time spent socializing with others.

Increased attention and time spent on healthcare/activities of daily living.

Adherence to a prescribed treatment program.

Adequate self-management of the Psychomotor Retardation.

A completed self-care (discharge) plan, including steps to be taken should the Psychomotor Retardation return or exacerbate.

Psychotic Thought/Behavior

Patient will verbalize:

Awareness of the presence of Psychotic Thought/Behavior.

Acceptance of responsibility for the presence of the Psychotic Thought/Behavior.

The precipitants for the Psychotic Thought/Behavior.

Warning signs that the Psychotic Thought/Behavior is exacerbating.

A plan of action to be taken should the Psychotic Thought/Behavior exacerbate.

Patient will demonstrate:

Absence of Psychotic Thought/Behavior for 72 hours.

Adherence to a prescribed treatment program.

Adequate management of the Psychotic Thought/Behavior.

Elimination of the Psychotic Thought/Behavior.

A completed self-care (discharge) plan, including steps to be taken should the Psychotic Thought/Behavior return or exacerbate.

Running Away

Patient will verbalize:

Acceptance of responsibility for the inability to manage urges to run away adequately.

The potential dangers of Running Away.

The adverse consequences of Running Away.

The precipitants for Running-Away behavior.

Alternative behaviors for Running Away.

Warning signs that the urge to run away is returning.

A plan of action to be taken should the urge to run away return.

Patient will demonstrate:

Adherence to a prescribed treatment program.

Control over the urge to run away without the use of one-to-one monitoring for 72 hours.

Ability to interrupt the urge to run away before it occurs.

A contingency plan for the Running-Away behavior.

Elimination of Running-Away behavior.

A completed self-care (discharge) plan, including steps to be taken should the urge to run away return.

Self-Mutilation

Patient will verbalize:

Acceptance of responsibility for Self-Mutilation behaviors.

The precipitants for Self-Mutilation urges.

Alternative actions to be implemented when feeling the urges to self-mutilate.

Warning signs that urges to self-mutilate are exacerbating.

A plan of action to be taken should the urges to self-mutilate exacerbate.

Patient will demonstrate:

Elimination of Self-Mutilation behaviors for 72 hours.

Adherence to a medication/treatment management program for Self-Mutilation.

Elimination of Self-Mutilation behaviors and urges.

A completed self-care (discharge) plan, including steps to be taken should the urges to self-mutilate return or exacerbate.

Sexual Trauma Perpetrator

Patient will verbalize:

The dangers of the rape or molestation behaviors.

The damaging consequences of rape or molestation behaviors.

Personal responsibility—rather than "blaming others"—for the rape or molestation behaviors.

A plan not to repeat rape or molestation behaviors.

Alternative behaviors for urges to rape or molest.

Warning signs that the urges to rape or molest are exacerbating.

A plan of action to be taken should the urges to rape or molest exacerbate.

Patient will demonstrate:

Adherence to a prescribed treatment program.

The capacity to verbalize anger rather than act on it.

The ability to interrupt traumatizing behaviors before they occur.

Elimination of the rape or molestation behaviors.

A completed self-care (discharge) plan, including steps to be taken should the urge to rape or molest return or exacerbate.

Substance Abuse

Patient will verbalize:

Acceptance of personal responsibility for the Substance Abuse.

The adverse impact of Substance Abuse and potential hazards of substance substitution.

The warning signs that the uncontrollable urge to abuse is returning.

A contingency plan of action to be taken should the urge to abuse persist.

A plan of action to be taken should a relapse occur.

Patient will demonstrate:

A written "Step One," which satisfactorily records the adverse impact of the Substance Abuse on the patient's and others' lives.

A three- to five-page paper that addresses Substance Abuse as a disease, the problems of substance substitution, the relapse indicators, and relapse avoidance techniques.

A written ongoing care plan for the Substance Abuse.

Implementation of the written personal care plan for the Substance Abuse.

Obtaining a 12-step program sponsor.

Abstinence from substances of abuse as evidenced by negative, random urine drug screenings.

Adherence to a medication/treatment program for the Substance Abuse.

A completed self-care (discharge) plan, including steps to be taken should a relapse occur.

Suicidal Thought/Behavior

Patient will verbalize:

Plans to harm oneself rather than act on them.

The precipitants for Suicidal Thought/Behavior.

Alternative actions to be taken when feeling suicidal.

Absence of suicidal thoughts.

Reasons for living.

Warning signs that Suicidal Thought/Behavior is exacerbating.

A plan of action to be taken should Suicidal Thought/Behavior exacerbate.

Patient will demonstrate:

Participation in a prescribed treatment program.

Adherence to a prescribed medication treatment program for the Suicidal Thought/Behavior.

Commitment to a behavioral contract not to harm oneself.

Elimination of Suicidal Thought/Behavior.

A completed self-care (discharge) plan, including steps to be taken should Suicidal Thought/Behavior return or exacerbate.

References

Altman LK: Oath as old as Apollo endures. The New York Times, May 15, 1990, B6

American Medical Association: Physicians' Current Procedural Terminology, CPT 1995. Chicago, IL, American Medical Association, 1994

American Medical Association: American Medical News 1994 Data Survey Summary. Chicago, IL, American Medical Association, 1995

American Psychiatric Association: Diagnostic and Statistical Manual of Mental Disorders, 3rd Edition. Washington, DC, American Psychiatric Association, 1980

American Psychiatric Association: Diagnostic and Statistical Manual of Mental Disorders, 3rd Edition, Revised. Washington, DC, American Psychiatric Association, 1987

American Psychiatric Association: Diagnostic and Statistical Manual of Mental Disorders, 4th Edition. Washington, DC, American Psychiatric Association, 1994

Angle HV, Cone JD, Hawkins RF, et al: Computer-assisted behavioral assessment, in Behavioral Assessment: New Directions in Clinical Psychology. Edited by Cone JD, Hawkins RF. New York, Brunner/Mazel, 1977, pp 35–84

Barlett DL, Steele JB: America: What Went Wrong. Kansas City, MO, Andrews & McMeel, 1992

Behar D, Rapoport JL, Berg CJ, et al: Computerized tomography and neuropsychological test measures in adolescents with obsessive-compulsive disorder. Am J Psychiatry 141:363–369, 1984

Brown J: The Quality Management Professional's Study Guide. Pasadena, CA, Managed Care Consultants, 1995

Brown SL: Family interviewing as a basis for clinical management, in The Family: Evaluation and Treatment. Edited by Hofling CK, Lewis JM. New York, Brunner/Mazel, 1980, pp 122–137

Colorado Department of Institutions, Division of Mental Health: Standards/rules and regulations for mental health centers and clinics. Denver, CO, Colorado Department of Institutions, March 1977

Congressional Budget Office: Congressional Budget Office 1994 Study. Washington, DC, Congressional Budget Office, 1995

Cooper H: Cost controls impel psych hospitals to establish more out-patient programs. The Wall Street Journal, March 16, 1994, sec 3, pp 1, 3

Darling v Charleston Community Memorial Hospital, 33 Ill 2d 326, 211 NE2d 253 (1965)

Donabedian A: Explorations in Quality Assessment and Monitoring, Vol 1: Definition of Quality and Approaches to Its Assessment. Ann Arbor, MI, Health Administration Press, 1980

Donabedian A: Explorations in Quality Assessment and Monitoring, Vol 2: The Criteria and Standards of Quality. Ann Arbor, MI, Health Administration Press, 1982

Drake DF: Reforming the Health Care Marketplace. Washington, DC, Georgetown University Press, 1994

Eddy DM: A Manual for Assessing Health Practices & Designing Practice Policies: The Explicit Approach. Philadelphia, PA, American College of Physicians, 1992

Elam v College Park Hospital, 132 Cal App 3d 322, 183 Cal Rptr 156 (1982)

Elkins R, Rapoport JL, Lipsky A: Obsessive-compulsive disorder of childhood and adolescence: a neurobiological viewpoint. Journal of the American Academy of Child Psychiatry 19:511–524, 1980

Ellwood PM: Shattuck lecture: outcomes management: a technology of patient experience. N Engl J Med 318:1549–1556, 1988

Federal Register: Medicare program: prospective payments for Medicare inpatient hospital services. Federal Register 48:39752–39890, 1983

Federal Register: Medicare program: prospective payment for Medicare final rule. Federal Register 49:234–340, 1984

Fetter RB, Shin Y, Freeman JL, et al: Construction of diagnosis-related groups. Med Care 18(2, suppl):5–20, 1980

Flannery J, Taylor G: Toward integrating psyche and soma: psychoanalysis and neurobiology. Can J Psychiatry 26:15–23, 1981

Flexner A: Medical Education in the United States and Canada: A Report to the Carnegie Foundation for the Advancement of Teaching. New York, The Carnegie Foundation, 1910

Foster Higgins: Survey of 2907 Employers. New York, Foster Higgins & Co, 1995

Geraty R: The latest generation of managed care: managed outcomes. Psychiatric Times, July 1994, p 61

Goodman D: Living at Light Speed. New York, Random House, 1994

Goold CP (ed): Hippocrates, Vol 1. London, Harvard University Press, 1995

Grant DE: America's economic outlaw: the U.S. health care system. Bull N Y Acad Med 55:20–24, 1994

Grant RL: The capacity of the psychiatric record to meet changing needs, in Psychiatric Records in Mental Health Care. Edited by Siegel C, Fischer SK. New York, Brunner/Mazel, 1981, pp 319–326

Gray B: The Profit Motive and Patient Care. Cambridge, MA, Harvard University Press, 1991

Grotstein JS, Solomon MF, Lang J (eds): The Borderline Patient. Hillsdale, NJ, Analytic Press, 1987

Healthcare Quality Improvement Act of 1986, PL No 99-60

Hearn E: Managing Medicaid. American Medical News, December 19, 1994, pp 13–16

Heilbrunn G: Biologic correlates of psychoanalytic concepts. J Am Psychoanal Assoc 27:597–626, 1979

Hoover CF, Insel TR: Families of origin in obsessive-compulsive disorder. J Nerv Ment Dis 172:207–215, 1984

InterQual: ISD-A Review System With Adult ISD Criteria. North Hampton, NH, 1993

Joint Commission on Accreditation of Healthcare Organizations: Accreditation Manual for Mental Health, Chemical Dependency, and Mental Retardation/Developmental Disabilities Services (1995 MHM), Vol 1: Standards. Oakbrook Terrace, IL, Joint Commission on Accreditation of Healthcare Organizations, 1994

Joint Commission on Accreditation of Healthcare Organizations: 1996 Comprehensive Accreditation Manual for Hospitals (CAMH). Oakbrook Terrace, IL, Joint Commission on Accreditation of Healthcare Organizations, 1995

Kiesler CA: Mental hospitals and alternative care. Am Psychol 37:349–360, 1982

Kim MJ, McFarland GK, McLane AM: Classification of Nursing Diagnoses. St. Louis, MO, CV Mosby, 1984

Longabaugh R, Fowler DR, Ryback R: The problem-oriented record in quality review, program planning and clinical research. International Journal of Mental Health 6:110–121, 1983

Marmor J: Psychoanalysis, psychiatry, and systems thinking. J Am Acad Psychoanal 10:337–350, 1982

Medical Records Institute: Toward an Electronic Patient Record. Newton, MA, Medical Records Institute, 1995

Medicare and Medicaid Patient and Program Protection Act of 1987, Amendment to Health Care Quality Improvement Act, sec 402, Pub L No 100-177

Meldman MJ, McFarland G, Johnson E: The Problem-Oriented Psychiatric Index and Treatment Plans. St. Louis, MO, CV Mosby, 1976

Meyersburg HA, Post RM: An holistic developmental view of neural and psychological processes: a neuro-biologic-psychoanalytic integration. Br J Psychiatry 135:139–155, 1979

National Committee for Quality Assurance: Health Plan Employer Data and Information Set (HEDIS 2.0 and 2.5). Washington, DC, National Committee for Quality Assurance, 1993/1995

Oss ME: Managed Behavioral Health Market Share in the United States, 1994. Gettysburg, PA, Behavioral Health Industry News, 1994

Othmer E, Othmer SC: The Clinical Interview Using DSM-III-R. Washington, DC, American Psychiatric Press, 1989

Parker S: Companies "carve-in" mental health care. Clinical Psychiatry News 23:1–2, 1995

Parloff MB: Psychotherapy research evidence and reimbursement decisions: Bambi meets Godzilla. Am J Psychiatry 139:718–727, 1982

Peer Review Improvement Act (Tax Equity and Fiscal Responsibility Act of 1982, Title I, Subtitle C, § 2142)

Problem-Oriented Medical Record Project: POMR: Self-Instruction for Practitioners. Chicago, IL, Michael Reese Hospital and Medical Center, 1978

Ryback RS, Longabaugh R, Fowler DR (eds): The Problem-Oriented Record in Psychiatry and Health Care. New York, Grune & Stratton, 1981

Social Security Amendments of 1972, Pub L No 92-603

Social Security Amendments of 1983, Pub L No 98-21

Taylor G: The emerging field of behavioral medicine. Perspectives in Psychiatry [University of Toronto, Department of Psychiatry] 4:1–5, 1985

Tax Equity and Fiscal Responsibility Act (TEFRA) of 1982, Pub L No 97-248

Transamerica Occidental Life: Medicare newsletter: documentation guidelines for evaluation and management (E/M) services. Transamerica Occidental Life, October 1994, pp 2–3

United Nations: United Nations 1994 Human Development Report. New York, United Nations, 1994

Vaillant GE, Perry JC: Personality disorders, in Comprehensive Textbook of Psychiatry-IV, 4th Edition, Vol 1. Edited by Kaplan HI, Sadock BJ. Baltimore, MD, Williams & Wilkins, 1985, pp 958–986

Weed LL: Medical Records, Medical Education and Patient Care. Cleveland, OH, Case Western Reserve University Press, 1969

Weil MM, Rosen LD: The technological revolution: psychiatry needs technology now. Psychiatric Times, September 1994, pp 37–39

World Health Organization: International Classification of Diseases, 9th Revision, Clinical Modification. Geneva, World Health Organization, 1980

Zimmerman M: Why are we rushing to publish DSM-IV? Arch Gen Psychiatry 45:1135–1138, 1988

Index

Page numbers printed in **boldface** *type refer to tables or figures.*